WORK**PLACE BULLYING** IN THE NHS

Workplace Bullying in the NHS

Edited by

Jacqueline Randle
Associate Professor
School of Nursing
University of Nottingham

Foreword by

Christine Webb

Radcliffe Publishing
Oxford • Seattle

Radcliffe Publishing Ltd
18 Marcham Road
Abingdon
Oxon OX14 1AA
United Kingdom

www.radcliffe-oxford.com
Electronic catalogue and worldwide online ordering facility.

British Library Cataloguing in Publication Data

A catalogue record for this book is available from the British Library.

ISBN-10 1 85775 783 1
ISBN-13 978 1 85775 783 5

Typeset by Advance Typesetting Ltd, Oxford
Printed and bound by TJ International Ltd, Padstow, Cornwall

This book is dedicated to my son, Samuel, and my husband, Matthew

Contents

Foreword

Whilst I am pleased to have the opportunity to write the foreword to *Workplace Bullying in the NHS*, I am sad that such a book is needed – and I can confirm that it *is* needed because I can recall many instances of bullying and poor responses to it from my career as a nurse, researcher and educator. Furthermore, my experience is that the same kinds of problems and failures arise in universities. This is not just in nursing departments – where it could be argued to be a 'contamination' of staff as a result of their previous NHS careers. On the contrary, bullying occurs across the board in universities and this was confirmed in a recent study of occupational stress in higher education in which I was involved as a researcher.[1]

Bullying sometimes takes the form of 'horizontal violence'[2] perpetrated among staff who are peers or are at similar levels in an organisation. For example, on my very first ward when I was just out of what was then called PTS, or Preliminary Training School, I was in the sluice taking hot and steaming bedpans from the boiler. The bedpans were heavy and difficult to manipulate with the large Cheatle forceps, and I paused to rest one on the edge of the boiler in order to get a better grip on it. A second-year student saw this and launched into a tirade about the bedpan no longer being sterile and insisted that I boil the whole lot again. I knew perfectly well that these bedpans were not meant to be sterile, but merely 'socially clean', and that I had done nothing wrong. But I was intimidated by this more senior student's behaviour towards me and so I said nothing and did as I was told.

I first heard the expression that nurses 'eat their young' several years ago in a speech about workforce bullying by Christine Hancock, then General Secretary of the UK Royal College of Nursing. This phrase certainly applied to me on many occasions during my nursing education and subsequent career, and is still relevant for nursing students and staff today, as this book shows.

At all stages of my clinical work I can recall incidents of this kind of intimidation and bullying by doctors of all positions from the most junior to the most senior. I am still haunted by my failure, when working as a clinical teacher with student nurses, to be assertive enough in relation to a surgical patient whose wound was leaking bile. I pointed this out to the surgical resident but he said that it was normal wound drainage and that I should know this. I was thus humiliated in front of the patient, my nursing student and other medical staff. I knew that the patient's anastomosis had broken down, but I was sufficiently undermined that I did not pursue the matter. When I met my student a couple of weeks later I asked her about the patient. She said that he was now back from the intensive care unit, having developed septicaemia and been returned to the operating theatre to have the anastomosis closed.

In another setting, as a more senior teacher, I was able to deal successfully with being bullied by a manager after confronting them in a prearranged meeting and asking a colleague to be present to support me. I had previously discussed the matter with a personnel officer, who therefore knew of problems in the department. However, although I was never threatened again, I was aware that several other people were having similar experiences and the personnel department allowed this situation to continue unchallenged. In my experience, if a manager seems to be 'delivering the goods' in their unit or department, then more senior managers are often prepared to turn a blind eye to what is going on.

As the contributors to this book and these personal examples illustrate, bullying is not 'just' an interpersonal matter but takes place in an organisational context that reinforces it by not taking action against it. The results are poor morale, a great deal of personal suffering, and staff sickness absence and turnover that are financially costly to the organisation. It is likely that patient care is also affected negatively by the ambience created by this bullying and lack of action to tackle it at its roots.

That I am not unique in being able to recall events of this kind throughout my career confirms that this book is relevant to the NHS work setting today. The various contributors give examples that are similar to mine and indeed, their illustrations go right across the board in terms of types, levels and possible ways of tackling the problem. Their concrete suggestions for actions are perhaps the most valuable part of what they offer, and the fact that there are now structures in place in many organisations to support staff shows that there is growing recognition of the extent of the problem. Whilst, as the contributors acknowledge, it will probably never be possible to eliminate bullying entirely from large organisations such as NHS trusts, the existence of anti-bullying policies and support facilities such as anti-bullying officers and employee assistance programmes should go a long way to helping individuals and groups of staff to make the workplace a more comfortable, productive and caring environment in which to work.

Christine Webb PhD, RN, FRCN
Professor of Health Studies, University of Plymouth
Executive Editor, *Journal of Advanced Nursing*
February 2006

References

1 Tytherleigh MY, Webb C, Cooper CL and Ricketts C. Occupational stress in UK higher education institutions: a comparative study of all staff categories. *Higher Education Research and Development*. 2005;24(1):41–61.
2 McKenna BG, Smith NA, Poole SJ and Coverdale JH. Horizontal violence: experiences of Registered Nurses in their first year of practice. *Journal of Advanced Nursing*. 2003;42:90–6.

Preface

Bullying is a sensitive issue. However, reports in the media and professional press suggest that bullying is no longer confined to the playground. The term 'bullying' is becoming more commonplace in the workplace but usually it is a term that is used loosely and indiscriminately from other negative behaviours. This encourages the myth that bullying is rife.

For the recipients of bullying, usually referred to as the victims, bullying cannot be underestimated. Victims may be coerced into reluctant resignation, enforced redundancy, early or ill health retirement. Healthcare workers who leave their jobs due to bullying can experience heavy drinking, eating disorders, panic attacks and nightmares. Similarly, the effects of bullying can result in a decrease in self-esteem and confidence, depression and stress. In extreme cases individuals may require psychiatric treatment. Usually the victim's family and friends are also affected.

Bullying not only affects the victim and their families but can also have an effect on healthcare teams as it can evoke feelings of anxiety, dismay, powerlessness and revenge. It can be very divisive, with team members being in an unenviable position. On the one hand they may feel they should be supporting the victim but at the same time they may actually like the bully and feel reluctant to oppose them. It is common for bullies to be socially undesirable to the victim, but to be extremely socially competent to others. As they are often socially intelligent, they are typically popular and may be very well liked by team members. It is also possible that individuals may fear that the bully could start victimising them.

Although the bully may be a certain 'personality type', current thinking is that it is the context of where we work that will influence whether bullying exists and is allowed to flourish. It is clear that the values and norms of the workplace influence how bullying is defined, how situations are interpreted, and whether bullying is recognised as a problem.

If we can accept that the context of the workplace influences behaviour, it could be that the NHS, like other large organisations, is characterised by circumstances that make bullying and harassment likely. These include organisational change and uncertainty, inadequate training, pressure from above, unrealistic targets and high stress levels. Changes such as downsizing, reorganisation in the workplace and top-down targets may exacerbate certain behaviours. As work organisations are increasingly changing and careers are insecure, this will ultimately impact on how people will treat each other, and bullying can actually serve an organisational purpose where it is a receptacle for projections of conflict and blame. The workplace culture may have bullying behaviour as a norm, and so people may be unwilling to challenge individual bullying behaviour that passively supports the bully.

If the values and norms of the workplace influence how bullying is defined in that context, how employees interpret situations and whether bullying is recognised as a problem, then we can assume that solutions can be implemented to limit the negative effects of bullying. This means that everyone within the workplace can contribute to the creation and maintenance of a bullying-free environment by changing. The best way to eliminate bullying in the workplace is to foster an environment that discourages bullying and ensures that everyone realises bullying is unacceptable. This means that as part of a team, you should ensure that colleagues know you will support them and that you see bullying as unacceptable. Team members are responsible for examining their own behaviour to ensure it does not cause problems, and those in senior positions are responsible for preventing incidents of bullying and reporting them immediately.

This will necessitate an understanding of the phenomenon, and as many people working in the NHS have been, and still are, victims of bullying, this book is written with the aim of providing remedies and solutions. Information provided in this book should help you be aware of the effects of bullying on an individual, colleagues, and even patients. From this awareness, solutions and strategies can be implemented in order to minimise the negative effects of bullying. This is aimed at different levels, whether it be organisational, professional or individual. We hope the information we provide will help you know what support you and your colleagues need.

Jacqueline Randle
January 2006

About the editor

Dr Jacqueline Randle qualified as a nurse in 1990 and worked as a staff nurse at Derriford Hospital in Plymouth. In 2000 she was awarded her PhD from Nottingham University. Since 1992 Jacqueline has worked in healthcare education, firstly at Plymouth University and for the last four years at the School of Nursing, University of Nottingham. She is an Associate Professor and works with pre-registration Masters of Nursing students and students studying at doctoral level. Jacqueline's research focus is healthcare education and she has been involved in a variety of funded projects, which enhance and develop students' learning. Her publications in books and professional journals focus on teaching and learning, and she has numerous publications that examine the phenomenon of workplace socialisation, self-esteem and bullying.

List of contributors

David Bullivent
NHS Management Consultant
Plymouth

Ian Grayling
Director of Short Courses
Life Long Learning Unit, University of Leicester

Dr Keith Hickling
Senior Lecturer
School of Nursing, University of Huddersfield

Cheryl Hume
Staff Nurse, Children's Services
Queen's Medical Centre, Nottingham

Malcolm Lewis
Senior Lecturer
Department of Health and Postgraduate Medicine, University of Central Lancashire

Dr Keith Stevenson
Deputy Director of Postgraduate Research Education
School of Nursing, University of Nottingham

Terry West
NHS Management Consultant
Plymouth

Chapter 1

Setting the scene

Jacqueline Randle

In order to help readers decide what bullying is and what it is not, this introductory chapter identifies the main themes relevant to bullying in the NHS. Bullying is a sensitive issue and usually attracts negative reactions, with many individuals, managers and NHS trusts choosing to ignore it or denying that it happens, hoping that it will go away. To do this is limiting, as the repercussions to individual health, the functioning of teams, systems and structures are far-reaching. Bullying does not only affect the individual, but it goes to the heart and the purpose of the NHS.[1]

Workplace bullying is increasingly being recognised as a serious problem in society and Field goes so far as to say that 'workplace bullying is ... the second greatest social evil after child abuse, with which it has many parallels'.[2] There is increasing evidence that the scale of bullying, harassment and violence towards healthcare staff is widespread.[3] Reports from the general media, published anecdotal evidence and results from surveys would suggest that workplace bullying is rife.

An issue worth pointing out early in the book is that bullying cannot be confined to an examination of the bully and the victim. This chapter will focus on the behaviour of the bully, but there is a wider picture, which will become clearer as you work through this book. Bullies do not operate in a vacuum. In focusing on bullies and victims, solutions can become too narrow, and a more comprehensive understanding is required. In order for the reader to arrive at this comprehensive understanding, definitions of workplace bullying are explored in more depth in Chapters 2 and 3, which allow the reader to understand the context of bullying in the framework of healthcare. Both of these chapters are based on extensive research studies and therefore offer a sound theoretical framework on which other chapters are based.

Once bullying has been recognised, it is important that it is tackled, and this may involve different levels of strategies. These strategies are identified in Chapter 4 by David Bullivent and Terry West, where practical solutions are offered to case studies of staff working in the NHS. In Chapter 5 we provide data and solutions for those working in healthcare education. This is important, as work suggests that this is where workplace bullying starts and students are often routinely bullied in order for them to successfully adopt the identity of the professional group. My earlier work also showed that students and nurses also bullied patients at times. This was extremely distressing to the students involved, but by the end of their training period, the majority of them had accepted that 'this is what happens'. To be able to challenge such ways of working, individuals need to be equipped with the appropriate skills and knowledge. Consequently, Chapter 6 by Ian Grayling and Keith Stevenson provides specific solutions and strategies aimed at the trainer/mentor. The final chapter, Chapter 7, by Keith Stevenson draws on the main themes apparent in this book and leads us towards the important conclusion, that the culture of the organisation plays a large part in whether bullying flourishes or diminishes. This is not to dismiss the part played by the individual bully or victim, but it does identify the need to take a macro-perspective on this phenomenon.

Key issues

In Chapter 2 you will be introduced to a thorough examination of definitions of bullying. For this introductory chapter it is enough to offer a commonly accepted and widely used definition. Adams describes bullying as 'the persistent, demeaning and downgrading of people through vicious words and cruel acts'.[4]

Bullying is generally characterised by three factors: intent, time duration and an imbalance of power. The problematic nature of these factors will be discussed in Chapter 3, but here it is worth mentioning that bullies often bully with intent and malice and may develop 'serial' bullying behaviours. The impact of bullying should not be underestimated. Those on the receiving end (commonly regarded as victims) may be coerced to resign, accept enforced redundancy or to take early or ill health retirement. Healthcare workers who leave their job because of bullying often experience heavy drinking, eating disorders, panic attacks, and nightmares.[5] Bullying often lowers self-esteem and victims often suffer from depression and stress.[6-11] Usually the victim's family and friends are also affected. Bullying has an effect on teams because it can evoke anxiety, dismay, powerlessness, and revenge.

Agreed definitions of bullying are still being debated but it is important to be able to recognise bullying behaviours.

What is bullying?

Please answer the following questions. Have you been:

- constantly criticised?
- ridiculed?
- undermined in front of others?
- sidelined or marginalised?
- made to feel vulnerable?
- treated differently?
- set unrealistic goals/work?
- denied information or knowledge necessary for you to achieve work objectives?
- denied support?
- given the 'silent treatment'?
- excessively monitored/supervised?

Have you had:

- your work/decisions dismissed, ignored or overruled?
- goalposts shifted without notice or reason?
- your work plagiarised/stolen or copied?
- responsibility removed from you and been given more menial jobs (without any legitimate reason for this to happen)?
- your authority removed/undermined?

If so it is likely that you have been bullied. These specific behaviours which characterise bullying are identified by Field and Quine amongst others.[2,12] Have you been on the receiving end of:

- destructive innuendo and sarcasm?
- verbal and non-verbal threats?
- inappropriate and hurtful jokes?
- physical violence?

Now ask yourself if you routinely display these types of behaviours to others. There is an important point here; you can be the victim and the bully simultaneously. It's easy to build a mental picture of the bully and the victim. The danger of these rigid stereotypes is that we begin to see the bully as nothing but a bully and the victim as nothing but a victim. But bullies can also be victims and victims can also be bullies.

Box 1.1 Scenario

Jeanette is a 36-year-old nurse who has been working as a senior staff nurse on a colorectal ward for five years.

On the morning ward round, in the presence of the multidisciplinary team, Jeanette's suggestions for pain management for a patient are ridiculed, and her request for additional pain relief medication is dismissed by the consultant surgeon. Jeanette has spent time with the patient assessing their pain needs and is surprised because she knows the surgeon agreed to pain relief in a similar patient. This is a characteristic of the relationship that exists between the surgeon and Jeanette, and Jeanette feels that the surgeon routinely picks on her and humiliates her.

When Jeanette asks why this decision was made, the surgeon fails to answer but instead asks Jeanette why the patient's wound dressing has not been changed. The surgeon then asks Jeanette to re-dress the patient's wound immediately, thus ensuring Jeanette is unable to continue on the ward round.

Has Jeanette been bullied? Whether or not Jeanette feels she has been bullied, this scenario demonstrates typical bullying behaviour.

- By overruling Jeanette's request in front of her colleagues and by publicly refusing her request, Jeanette is being undermined.
- By not automatically explaining why the request has been refused, Jeanette is being denied information.
- By refusing Jeanette's request for pain relief but granting other patients' requests, the consultant may make Jeanette feel ostracised.
- By requesting that Jeanette focuses on another aspect of work, the consultant forces Jeanette to step away from her responsibilities of the ward round for a task that a colleague could have performed.

Bullies undermine individuals, especially in front of others. They express doubts about a person's performance or standard of work without substantive and quantifiable evidence. They may constantly criticise or ridicule achievements.

Another typical behaviour is ostracising the victim, making them more vulnerable and easier to control and subjugate. Individuals who bully single out and treat individuals differently. For example, nursing staff may go for a coffee break together, always leaving the same healthcare assistant to cope on her own with patients.

Why does bullying happen?

Bullies are often perceived as dysfunctional or as having a psychopathic personality.[2] The victims are similarly perceived as being non-assertive, avoiding conflict, shy, and making little effort to integrate into work. They are also more prone to anxiety and depression.[13] The concept of the personality type is discussed in much more depth in Chapters 3 and 4, and here there is an explanation of why a more comprehensive approach than personality types is required.

Part of this comprehensive approach is the notion that the workplace environment influences behaviour. The majority of this book acknowledges this fact, and a lot of the solutions we offer are aimed at an organisational level. The theoretical explanation is that in the NHS, like any organisation, it is often work conditions that trigger bullying and harassment.[14] These include:

- organisational change and uncertainty
- inadequate training
- pressure from above
- unrealistic targets
- high stress levels.

If you look at the above list it is easy to see how changes such as downsizing, reorganisation, and top-down targets may exacerbate certain behaviours. Changes within organisations and the fact that jobs are now less secure will ultimately impact on how people treat each other. However, not all people in the NHS go on to bully, so it may be that we cannot reject personality factors altogether. The values and norms of the workplace do, however, influence how bullying is defined in that context, how employees interpret situations, and whether bullying is recognised as a problem.

Box 1.2 Key points

- The term 'bullying' is used loosely and often borrowed indiscriminately from other negative activities, such as racial or sexual harassment.
- Bullying is difficult to define and evaluate accurately.
- Different groups can interpret bullying in different ways. What a trade union may perceive as bullying, an employer may perceive as a change in policy or management.
- It is easy to build a mental picture of the bully and the victim. The danger of these rigid stereotypes is that we begin to see the bully as nothing but a bully, and the victim as nothing but a victim. But bullies can also be victims and victims can also be bullies.
- Accusing someone of bullying can be detrimental to the alleged bully (if they are not aware of the effect of their actions) and to the victim (if it causes the bullying to worsen).

References

1　Madge T. Where next for the NHS? *Nursing Standard*. 2003;17:3.
2　Field T. *Bully in Sight*. Wantage, Oxfordshire: Success Unlimited; 1996.
3　UNISON (2003) *Bullying at Work*. www.unison.org.uk/acrobat/13375.pdf (accessed 30 November 2005).
4　Adams A. *Bullying at Work – how to confront and overcome it*. London: Virago Press; 1992.
5　Doherty K. High cost of bullying to nurses and trusts revealed [News]. *Nursing Standard*. 2003;17:7.
6　Reeve J. *Past caring? A longitudinal study of the modes of change in the professional self-concept and global self-concepts of students undertaking a three year Diploma in Nursing course* (unpublished PhD dissertation). Nottingham: University of Nottingham; 2000.
7　Randle J. The effect of a three year pre-registration training course on students' self-esteem. *Journal of Clinical Nursing*. 2001;10:293–300.
8　Randle J. Past caring: the influence of technology. *Nursing Education in Practice*. 2001;1:157–65.
9　Randle J. Bullying in the nursing profession. *Journal of Advanced Nursing*. 2003;43:395–401.
10　Randle J. Changes in self-esteem during a 3 year pre-registration Diploma in Higher Education (Nursing) programme. *Journal of Clinical Nursing*. 2003;12:142–3.
11　Thompson DA. *Bullying: effective strategies for long term improvement*. London: Routledge Falmer; 2002.
12　Quine L. Workplace bullying in nurses. *Journal of Health Psychology*. 2001;6:73–84.
13　Einarsen S and Skogstad A. Bullying at work: epidemiological findings in public and private organisations. *European Journal of Work and Organisational Psychology*. 1996;5:185–201.
14　Sullivan C, cited by Parish C. Bullying can have a negative effect on clinical outcomes. *Nursing Standard*. 2003;17:4–5.

Chapter 2

Workplace bullying

Keith Hickling

Introduction

Any individual who experiences workplace bullying, either as a 'victim' or as an observer, is left puzzled and confused as to how this happens.

> Why is this happening to me? What kind of work situation have I found myself in that creates acts of harassment and bullying? How can I protect myself or my colleagues? Can I continue to work in such a situation? Is there something wrong with me?

These are the kind of questions that you might ask in such a situation. As professionals we may have formed preconceptions about the working environment. We may have expectations of mutual respect, co-operation, teamwork and skilled leadership that can be shattered by the experience of workplace bullying. As with many stressful situations, our emotions can cloud our critical and analytical judgement, and we may feel lost, persecuted, distressed, angry or depressed.

Generally we may feel powerless, and this is often the key component of our response to the experience of bullying. However, we are not powerless; we can understand the phenomenon from an educated and informed position, based upon the established research. This means we can act – as managers we can take steps to reduce bullying, as members of the team we can act, individually and collectively, to change a bullying culture.

As professionals we have all studied hard to understand our professional roles. Evidence-based practice is central to continued improvement and excellence in professional practice, in the NHS, in schools, in universities, in the emergency services and in businesses.

This chapter will consider the evidence related to workplace bullying. What is it, and how can we understand its 'causes'? Can we understand the context and, more importantly, can we make changes that reduce the incidence of workplace bullying? What is the relationship between workplace bullying, stress at work and job satisfaction?

I will begin by taking a position related to how environments can engender and sustain acts of bullying. Can we understand bullying based more upon discrete behaviours rather than seeking to understand the 'pathology' of the bully? Finally we will consider an action plan for dealing with workplace bullying based on published research. Alongside this we will consider the legislative framework in the UK, and ask whether these changes provide a context for attitude change related to work environments.

The chapter will be divided into four sections. Firstly, I will state the learning outcomes. I will then provide a section of reading. Following this will be a reflective discussion and finally a 'respond' section that poses questions and possible actions that could help you deal with workplace bullying.

After reading this chapter you should be able to:

- appreciate the complexities of the phenomenon of workplace bullying based upon the research
- form your own conclusions as to whether we can understand the environmental factors that relate to the presence of workplace bullying
- form an action plan, as a manager or as a member of the team, in order to tackle workplace bullying or to prevent it
- assist colleagues to deal with the effects of workplace bullying.

Background

The modern history of our understanding of workplace bullying can be seen as beginning with Andrea Adams' book *Bullying at Work*, published in 1992.[1] While more recent research has refined the positions that Andrea Adams outlined, her position remains valid in many ways. A great deal of research has been conducted since 1992.

While it is dangerous to over-simplify the history of workplace bullying research, we could see it passing through the following stages:

1 concentration on the nature of the *'bully'*
2 examination of the dynamics involved with *'victims'*
3 examination of organisational context and culture.

The definitional question

Starting with definitions can be dangerous, as it may colour further examination of the phenomenon. However, I feel that in this case it is beneficial as it quite graphically illustrates the problems of understanding bullying.

Early definitions: false trails?

In 1992, Andrea Adams defined workplace bullying as follows:[1]

> Persistent criticism and personal abuse in public or private, which humiliates and demeans the person.

Her position would appear to be 'anti-bully' and 'pro-victim'. In her book, these two labels are value laden and carry with them the potential to blame the bullies for the whole workplace bullying problem. Adams established her position based upon the view that there are two forms of human aggression.[2] One form has the aim to damage or to harm; the other form is a self-assertive aggression, which merely facilitates the pursuit of a goal.

There are benefits in developing assertiveness: benefits where bullies learn to be assertive rather than aggressive; and benefits where victims learn to be assertive rather than passive. However, Adams' position is based upon understanding workplace bullying as merely a form of human aggression and thus it is essentially bully blaming.[1]

In 1996, Tim Field defined bullying at work in the following manner:[3]

> Bullying consists of:
> - refusal to recognise, face up to, tackle and overcome one's own weaknesses, failings and shortcomings
> - denial of responsibility for the consequences of one's own actions and behaviours on others.
>
> If the bully is in a position of management, control, trust, etc., then also:
> - refusal to accept the legal and moral obligation for the safety, care and well-being of the person(s) in their charge.

This definition requires some consideration, as it moves from a far more extreme position on causation and solutions. In profiling the bully, Field builds a personality profile and introduces the notion of the psychopathic personality.[3] While he does not say that all bullies are psychopathic, the impression in his work is that there is a close association between the two. He even suggests that this is a result of 'brain malfunction' or right brain hemisphere syndrome, which he does not explain.

Thus the central position in the early years of theorising about workplace bullying takes an unfortunate direction. While there may be some individuals with anti-social personality disorder (psychopaths) who may appear in the workplace, there is no evidence that this is very common.

Before leaving Adams' and Field's work, it is worth noting that the Andrea Adams Trust and Tim Field's work have both assisted and supported a large number of victims of workplace bullying. While definitional discussions are important, the work of these individuals and organisations must be recognised.

The question of intent

Field also introduced the issue of the intent of the bully into the debate. He states:[3]

> The intent of the behaviour is to demean and to belittle in order to gratify the self.

Later in 1997, Peter Randall adds:[4]

> Bullying is the aggressive behaviour arising from the deliberate intent to cause physical or psychological distress to others.

It is worth considering this position for a moment. This position reinforces the bully-blaming stance. The dangers in this position are that managers and members of the team may be led to look no further than finding and blaming the bully. This may have the effect of conveniently finding the scapegoat bully and failing to consider other factors. While in some rare cases an individual bully may be the sole cause, in most cases, there are other factors. Later when we consider the bully–victim relationship, we will see that victims can also become bullies.

The question of intent, I would argue, is another false trail in understanding workplace bullying. Indeed, any solicitor will tell you how difficult it is to establish intent. Therefore finding the bully and proving the intent would not offer a solution to many situations where workplace bullying is occurring.

Bully–victim dyads

If we cannot understand workplace bullying merely as a problem of psychopathic bullies, and if there is a problem of the intentional acts of bullies, can we understand workplace bullying as a product of the dynamics between bullies and their victims?

Moving towards organisational context

Einarsen and Skogstad have provided an objective overview of published research regarding the causes of bullying.[5] They examine the literature related to personality traits and bullying. Previous research has suggested that the victim's personality may be a factor in the dynamics of workplace bullying.[6,7]

The 'victim' personality has been described as characterised by having low self-esteem, social anxiety, and over-conscientiousness. Indeed, some have suggested that some victims may act as 'provocative' victims as a result of these character-istics.[8] Felson has also suggested that victims may also violate social norms, thus eliciting aggressive behaviour in others.[9]

In contrast, bullies have variously been described as having an authoritarian or abrasive personality, having a background as a schoolyard bully, acting as a petty tyrant, or possibly having a proclivity for sexual harassment.[8] However, there is some evidence that victims can become bullies.

The research into the characteristics of bullies and their victims and into the dynamics of the dyadic relationship will continue. My view is that this research is important to our understanding of workplace bullying, while we have to take care not to allow this to become 'victim blaming'. However, understanding workplace bullying requires an even wider perspective and this has been provided based upon Scandinavian research.

The organisational context

Einarsen and Skogstad suggest that the model of workplace bullying that has received the most attention in Scandinavia is the position that particular work environments may engender, foster or sustain workplace bullying.[5]

Einarsen and Skogstad have provided a very useful overview of the broader factors affecting workplace bullying which they outline as follows:[5]

- personality traits of victims and bullies
- inherent characteristics of human interaction in organisations
- factors associated with particular work environments and conditions.

Thus we can see that Scandinavian research presents a broad position based on a complex relationship between organisational and social factors, while accepting that personality factors contribute to the occurrence of workplace bullying.

Based upon this position, Einarsen moves to a broader definition of workplace bullying:[10]

> ... a person is bullied or harassed when he or she is repeatedly subjected to negative acts in a situation where the victim finds it difficult to defend himself/herself. (p. 9)

Einarsen here provides a significant improvement in defining workplace bullying. No mention of intent and no 'bully blaming'. Indeed Einarsen provides a new framework for a more objective approach to measuring the incidence of workplace bullying, along with a means of defining more precisely the specific kinds of acts that constitute bullying (of which there will be more later).

From this information, we have been developing a model of workplace bullying that is more comprehensive. The model incorporates a number of personal, organisational and social dimensions that interact to produce the bullying acts and these in turn produce effects on individual(s).

The model may be presented as shown in Figure 2.1.

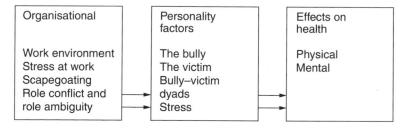

Figure 2.1 A summary of theoretical positions on workplace bullying.

You will note the inclusion of some new terms here. These illustrate the relationship between the Scandinavian approach to workplace bullying and its relationship to other research into the dynamics of the workplace.

Leymann has argued that personality factors are irrelevant to the study of bullying and that the primary cause of workplace bullying is the environment and working conditions.[11] Brodsky sees work pressures as a key concept in understanding the occurrence of workplace bullying.[7] Kahn *et al.* have associated role ambiguity and role conflict with stress at work,[12] and Einarsen and Skogstad have linked workplace bullying with both stress at work and high levels of role ambiguity and role conflict.[5]

Thus we have an emerging association between workplace bullying, work stress and high levels of two phenomena long used to measure work environments – namely role conflict and role ambiguity. It is important to note that here we are not dealing with causal relationships (although some authors may claim such). Here we are dealing with correlations. With correlations we may see high levels of stress correlated with high role conflict and high role ambiguity; these high levels may also correlate with a high incidence of workplace bullying. These relationships are not causal; we cannot yet prove that one factor 'causes' the other to increase. These factors may merely be interrelated or they may be affected by another, as yet unknown, factor. Alternatively we may never find a causal relationship.

However, this does not mean that we should ignore such research – social and psychological research is often concerned with correlations. The utility of the research for managers and team members lies in the associations. In simple terms, affecting organisational, cultural and social factors in the workplace can reduce the incidence of workplace bullying (again this will be discussed in more detail later).

Einarsen's theoretical framework on workplace bullying is presented in diagrammatic form in Figure 2.2.[10] Interestingly, Einarsen and Skogstad conclude their discussion by suggesting that harassment may in itself be an inherent characteristic of human interaction in organisations or it may be the potential outcome of some of the many conflicts that inevitably exist in organisations.[5] This does not mean that workplace bullying is inevitable and that nothing organisations or individuals do can prevent this. Rather, recognising this inherent tendency towards conflict is essential in preventing workplace bullying.

Box 2.1 Summary: taking stock

Following Andrea Adams' publication of her book *Bullying at Work* in 1992 we have seen the development of an increasingly sophisticated understanding of the phenomenon of workplace bullying. From early 'bully blaming' we have moved towards a more sophisticated understanding of the relationship between bullies and victims. Einarsen's position incorporates interpersonal, intrapersonal, cultural, social and organisational factors.

We also see the development of a sophisticated understanding of the relationship between workplace bullying, high levels of work stress and high levels of role conflict and role ambiguity as expressed in studies of specific work teams.

Role conflict and role ambiguity

It is worthwhile for us to pause for a moment and examine these factors. Role conflict is defined as the conflict between the needs and expectations of different roles, particularly as these are related to work stress.[13] Role conflict can occur between work roles and family and social roles. For example, work–family conflict is greater when children are under school age or when wives are employed in managerial or professional roles.[13] Recent focus by health promoters and politicians upon work–life balance illustrates the concerns in this area.

Psychologists have studied the relationship between role conflict and stress over many years, and measures of role conflict are well established. The relationship between role conflict and work stress is unclear; clearer relationships can be established between role conflict and job satisfaction. However, some researchers have established relationships between role conflict and physiological stress, and with negative health outcomes such as coronary heart disease.[12,14,15]

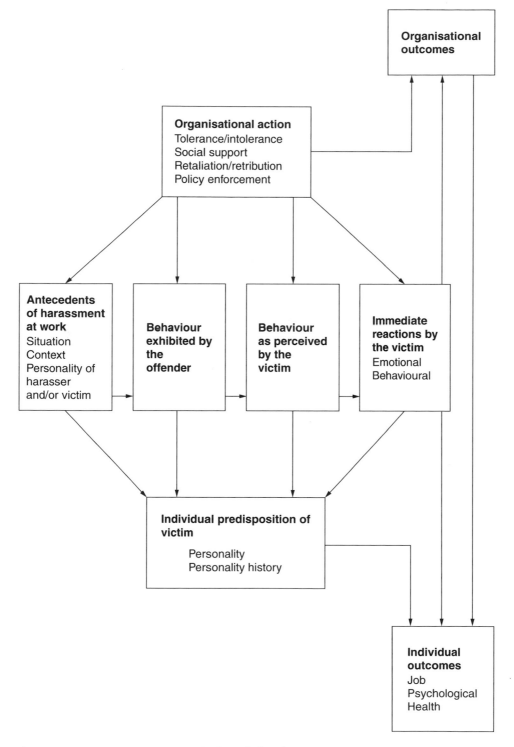

Figure 2.2 A theoretical framework of workplace bullying.

Kahn has identified four types of role conflict:[16]

1 *intra-sender conflict*: different prescriptions and proscriptions from a colleague may be incompatible
2 *inter-sender conflict*: pressures from one person oppose pressures from another person
3 *inter-role conflict*: membership in one organisation is in conflict with membership of other groups
4 *person–role conflict*: where role requirements violate moral values, or needs and aspirations lead to behaviours unacceptable to one's colleagues.

Thus role conflict can occur as a worker attempts to match work roles with social and family roles, but may also occur within work roles. For example, if a newly appointed ward manager has been promoted from within the nursing team, she/he may find that their person–role conflict may become apparent as they adjust to reconciling previous peer friendships with the new leadership and management role. In any team situation, mixed messages may produce inter-sender conflict, as team members send different or even opposing messages related to role expectations to colleagues. A classic case in the NHS is the conflict between professional standards of patient care and the pressures and constraints of dealing with difficult day-to-day decisions often constrained by tight resources and staffing shortages. Thus the professional role and the financial management role may conflict.

It is not difficult to see how high levels of role conflict could contribute to increased work stress. It is also possible to imagine how high levels of role conflict may increase the incidence and experience of workplace bullying. However, let us be cautious here; we are not yet able to argue for causal links in either direction. We merely see a correlation, we have no means of knowing whether some aspect of emergent bullying behaviours contributes to high role conflict or whether high role conflict in the workplace fosters and sustains bullying behaviours.

While role conflict relates to conflicts *between* roles, such as family and community roles versus professional roles; or role conflict *within* roles such as those conflicts evident in the role of colleague versus line manager, role ambiguity is subtly different.

Role ambiguity, which is strongly related to role conflict, relates to uncertainty about specific job roles. This may relate to the extent of your authority and responsibilities, and the way in which your work is evaluated.[13] Adequacy of training is related to this possible stressor, as is the quality of communications in the organisation. This can be related to harassment where there is deliberate withholding or distortion of information.[17]

An example of role ambiguity may be seen where a manager is given a task to complete within a team and there are mixed signals related to authority and responsibility. If the senior manager says 'you're responsible, I trust you, get on with it' but then constantly interferes and undermines the manager, then role ambiguity is engendered.

Szilagyi *et al.* suggest that higher levels of role ambiguity and role conflict are associated with low levels of job satisfaction,[18] while Bedeian and Armenakis found that both role ambiguity and role conflict had an effect upon job-induced tension, and this in turn affected job satisfaction.[19]

Therefore in summary I am suggesting the following points of review:

- understanding workplace bullying is complex and includes levels of individual, interpersonal, social and professional group and organisational behaviours, expectations and cultures
- workplace bullying can be seen as correlated with other work factors such as work stress and measures of role conflict and role ambiguity.

Measuring workplace bullying

There are many ways to attempt to measure workplace bullying. A researcher could, for example, merely ask 'Have you ever been bullied at work or witnessed a colleague being bullied at work?'. However, as we have seen this can be problematic. How do we understand what constitutes workplace bullying? Can we agree definitions? If a researcher attempts to define workplace bullying, can this attempt further bias the response?

Clearly this bias could occur. A great deal of research into workplace bullying has been conducted by the trade unions, UNISON, the Royal College of Nursing (RCN) and the Manufacturing Science and Finance Union (MSF), and other trade unions have conducted studies and presented their conclusions, which are often based on incidents of workplace bullying, whether they be experienced or witnessed. These research projects are very important in raising awareness of the problem, and often in acquainting members of staff with levels of support for victims. Indeed, the workplace bullying agenda, arguably, would not have moved forward at the pace that it has done without the campaigning of trade unions.

However, there are some issues related to this kind of research that we would need to consider in evaluating its usefulness. In addition to the problems of the lack of shared understanding of what constitutes workplace bullying, there is the further problem of response bias. If my line manager asks me whether I've ever been bullied at work I may make a certain kind of response to him. If my trade union asks me the same question, perhaps in a written questionnaire or on email, I could respond very differently. Indeed, I may feel that in order to assist my trade union in highlighting the particular problem, and in supporting my colleagues who may be victims of workplace bullying, I ought to reconsider that little incident last month and classify this as workplace bullying and respond accordingly.

There is also the problem of a self-selecting response. If I have been bullied at work or have witnessed a colleague being bullied I am more likely to respond to the questionnaire. Therefore if 50% of trade union members answer the questionnaire it may be possible for 80–90% of these to report workplace bullying simply because they become a self-selecting group.

Since a great deal of the research is based in organisations or organised by trade unions targeting a professional group, we need to deal with reported incidence figures carefully. The words 'harassment' or 'bullying' are also very value loaded and this could affect responses in either direction. Einarsen has led the way towards a more objective measurement of the phenomenon.

Einarsen and negative acts

Einarsen has developed an approach to measuring workplace bullying that avoids some of the pitfalls of some research. Einarsen avoids using these words by using a discrete scale of 'negative acts' and asking respondents to report whether they have experienced these.

In a study of male employees in the Norwegian marine engineering industry, Einarsen and Raknes developed the scale, which measures harassment (workplace bullying) through a Negative Acts Questionnaire (NAQ).[6] The criteria are based upon categories derived from previously published literature on workplace bullying.[7,20] Depth interviews were also conducted with victims of harassment in order to further validate these behavioural categories.

Their research revealed that 88.5% of respondents (all males in the sample) had experienced at least one of the behaviours measured by the NAQ scale over the past six months. Most frequently endorsed items were 'Someone withholding information so that your work gets complicated' (55.7%) and 'Neglect of your opinion or views' (53.6%). Endorsement levels for all other items were relatively high (between 18% and 48%).[17] Examination of the age profile of the respondents revealed that men aged above 50 years experienced significantly fewer negative acts then men below 40 years; overall younger men reported significantly more negative behaviours than older men.

Behavioural measures of negative acts were listed follows:[17]

1 someone withholding necessary information so that your work gets complicated
2 unwanted sexual advances
3 ridicule or insulting teasing
4 being ordered to work below your level of competence
5 being deprived of responsibility for work tasks
6 gossip or rumours about you
7 social exclusion from co-workers or work group activities
8 repeated offensive remarks about you or your private life
9 verbal abuse
10 unwanted sexual attention
11 hints or signals from others that you should quit your job
12 physical abuse or threats of physical abuse
13 repeated reminders about your blunders
14 silence or hostility as a response to your questions or attempts at conversations
15 devaluing your work or your efforts
16 neglect of your opinions or views
17 offending telephone calls or written messages
18 'funny' surprises
19 devaluing of your 'rights' and opinions with reference to your gender
20 devaluing of your 'rights' and opinions with reference to your age
21 exploitation at work, such as private errands
22 reaction from others because you work too hard.

The NAQ measure was also compared with a Work Environment measure and a measure of psychological health. Einarsen and Raknes found significant correlations between experience of negative acts (NAQ) and both psychological health and job satisfaction.[17] This research focused upon the experience of male workers in the Norwegian marine engineering industry and has established links between experience of negative acts (bullying), work environments and general mental health.

Einarsen and Raknes utilised a 36-item work satisfaction questionnaire developed by O'Brien *et al.* and extended by Marek *et al.*[17,21,22] These work satisfaction measures were grouped around six factors. Einarsen and Raknes found that non-violent harassment and bullying were correlated with low job satisfaction.[17] Work-related harassment was strongly connected with dissatisfaction with supervision and leadership, whereas personal derogation and social exclusion were associated with strong dissatisfaction with co-worker interactions. They also found that reported experience of harassment was higher among younger men.

Einarsen *et al.* also studied harassment by surveying 4200 members of six different labour unions.[6] In this study they used a measure of role conflict and role ambiguity developed by Rizzo *et al.*,[23] and found correlations between high incidence of bullying and high measures of role conflict and role ambiguity.

It seems that workplace bullying appears to co-exist with high stress and high role conflict and role ambiguity, with negative effects of staff satisfaction. Whatever the cause–effect relationships are, it seems that we cannot ignore its negative effects on staff health. We also see research developing a clearer means of identifying discrete behaviours that together represent a picture of workplace bullying. These allow managers and staff to identify the means to tackle the problem.

Reflect

Based upon your reading of the discussion above, we can now apply your understanding to specific aspects of your workplace. Read the exercises below and ask yourself the questions raised. When you have completed these exercises move on to the 'Respond' section.

Exercise one

Here is a list of types of bullying acts as described by Peter Randall.[4] Consider these and ask yourself:

1 do I agree that these categories represent workplace bullying?
2 have I ever experienced or witnessed these behaviours?

Examples of harassment[4]

- Remarks, derogatory comments, jokes
- Offensive or suggestive literature, e.g. pin-ups, racist jokes
- Unwanted physical contact
- Physical or verbal assault
- Unwelcome sexual advances
- Coercing sexual intercourse
- Embarrassing, threatening, humiliating, patronising or intimidating remarks
- Unwarranted threats of disciplinary action
- Undermining a person's esteem

- Unacceptable aggressive style from supervisor/manager
- Suggestive remarks
- Insulting behaviour or gestures

Consider
There are some difficult categories here. For example, 'remarks' and 'jokes'. Humour is important in the workplace, but you may consider situations where jokes get out of hand and become derogatory, insulting and demeaning. Bullies can hide behind humour as an excuse to harass others.

Exercise two

You are asked as either the team manager or as a member of the team to 'audit' your working environment and report whether these aspects of the working environment exist in your area.
   Ask the following questions:

1 how likely is it that these will be evident in your workplace?
2 do you consider that these represent an 'unacceptable culture' related to workplace bullying?

Unacceptable culture[4]

- Pin-ups, 'girlie' calendars on notice boards or desks
- General bantering across offices
- Making one particular employee the target of jokes
- Loud personal comments about or to colleagues
- Common use of offensive language or suggestive comments
- Aggressive style of management

Consider
Again there are some difficult categories here. 'General bantering across offices' often exists, but where is the fine line between supportive banter and bullying? How does your workplace culture handle situations where individuals object to this kind of culture?

Respond

How does one respond to this information on workplace bullying? I will divide this section into four parts:

1 *managers*: what to do to prevent workplace bullying
2 *staff*: what to do to prevent workplace bullying
3 *managers*: what to do when you encounter workplace bullying
4 *staff*: what to do when you encounter workplace bullying.

Managers: what to do to prevent workplace bullying

Prevention is better than having to deal with the problem. Creating an atmosphere of respect and tolerance takes time and effort. Being aware of the 'difference' triggers that might lead to workplace bullying is important. These may be factors such as gender, race, disability, religion or age but may also be something simply related to someone being shy.

- Use opportunities to talk to staff about the issue of workplace bullying; the problem hides in the shadows and a real dialogue with staff is the best form of prevention. Show by example that you do not resort to bullying and threats. This does not mean that you cannot manage – good management skills are completely devoid of bullying. Difficult situations such as dealing with poor staff performance or even misconduct can be handled without resorting to bullying.
- Demonstrate your tolerance of difference; more than this, demonstrate that you welcome difference and that the team is stronger because of the positive contribution of diversity. Be careful around the use of humour; be aware that it can soon stray into intimidation, ridicule and workplace bullying.
- If approached by staff with questions or complaints, be objective – as you have seen, situations can be wrongly labelled as workplace bullying. However, be aware that real situations can arise, and staff need support if making a complaint.
- Organisational procedures can be used to bully staff. So take advice if you are unsure about the use of a procedure, and always check yourself in your application of procedures in relation to fairness and equity. If respect, dignity and objectivity are always present in your practices, even when you may be involved in disciplinary action applied to a member of your staff, these difficult situations can be handled professionally and with equity and fairness.
- Get to know the law as it relates to the workplace. Legislation on discrimination on the grounds of gender, race, disability, religion and age is not only vital to your work as a manager, but also the principles contained in these approaches to 'human rights' and 'dignity at work' can inform all interactions at work (see discussion later in this chapter).

Staff: what to do to prevent workplace bullying

The most important point is to avoid labelling situations as workplace bullying when they are not. As with the word 'stress', we tend to overuse terms like 'bullying', 'harassment' or 'bully'. While these can provide useful labels for our understanding of the world of work, we need to use these with caution.

- Do your homework – get to know the law as it relates to the workplace. You need to understand the legislation on discrimination on the grounds of gender, race, disability, religion and age. Responsibilities do not only apply to managers; all citizens and workers are bound by these laws. Not only should you avoid any situations where you might be drawn to resort to workplace bullying and thus become discriminatory in your working practice, but also it is only on the basis that all workers respect others' 'human rights' and the right to 'dignity at work' that we can prevent workplace bullying.
- Examine your organisation's policy on 'harassment at work' and all the related organisational information related to equality and diversity. Talk about the issue;

these problems can thrive on our reluctance to talk about these sometimes difficult issues. Joining a trade union or participating in equal opportunities working parties can also assist you to protect yourself and others. Talk openly with your manager and raise the issue of prevention of workplace bullying at staff meetings.

- If approached by a colleague who feels that they are being bullied, be supportive, share information that you have, and encourage your colleague to report the matter. Remember that good procedures on harassment at work are couched in terms of the member of staff approaching the alleged bully, perhaps with the support of a harassment advisor, saying what the behaviours are that are objectionable and asking very firmly for these to stop. In most cases this resolves the matter; in rare cases the matter may need to be taken further.

Managers: what to do when you encounter workplace bullying

All reports and accusations of workplace bullying need to be taken seriously. It takes great courage to report these matters and staff are often distressed and afraid. Make it clear that you do not condone workplace bullying.

- Check your organisational procedures and take advice from personnel or human resources. Take advice from a senior colleague. Give time for the person making the complaint to consider their possible actions. Advise them to see a harassment advisor if your organisation has these. Be careful not to act hastily; in most cases, moving in a more considered way and not acting immediately is better. In extreme cases, where a physical or sexual assault has taken place or where these are clearly threatened, you need to act immediately, and again you would obviously take advice from your manager and from personnel professionals.
- If a harassment advisor or a trade union representative is involved, treat their involvement positively; they are there to assist and support. Remember there is a risk to you and to your organisation if you fail to act appropriately. You have clear responsibilities with respect to a number of pieces of legislation, and failure to act may lead to a legal challenge against your organisation or against you personally.
- If you are accused of workplace bullying by a member of staff, treat the complaint seriously and objectively. The label is sometimes misused and the complaint may be based on a misunderstanding. However, be prepared to learn from the experience, no matter how negative this may feel initially. We all make mistakes and say the wrong thing sometimes. If these accusations are serious, then take advice from your manager and from personnel. Vexatious complaints do occur, but be aware that you may have acted wrongly. The main position that you need to maintain is that if you have acted wrongly you are willing to stop this behaviour and apologise.

Staff: what to do when you encounter workplace bullying

If you experience workplace bullying as a victim this can be very disconcerting. The victim feels threatened, scared and angry.

- Get help immediately. In extreme cases you may be injured or the victim of a criminal offence. Get help and report the matter to the police. No one can be expected to tolerate physical or sexual assault in the workplace. Along with police involvement you will need the support of friends and family, possibly your trade union, and certainly your organisation's human resources department. Although you may feel that the situation is impossible and that you may not have a positive view of your future and your continued employment, with support you will find your way through this and rebuild your confidence.

- Many acts of workplace bullying are, however, much more subtle. Psychological bullying includes the use of threats, innuendo, distorted humour and unwarranted criticism and pressure. The impact of these techniques is more insidious, and you may become overly self-critical and even depressed during this time.

- The best techniques here are to be assertive and immediately object to these bullying behaviours, either in private or in public. However, sometimes you may be shocked and miss this opportunity. If you have the confidence, approach the bully as soon as possible and point out that these behaviours were offensive, that you felt harassed or bullied and that you want these behaviours to stop.

- If the bully refuses to accept or subsequently continues the bullying behaviour then seek assistance and advice from your line manager, a harassment advisor, personnel advisors or a trade union representative. Talk to your friends about the matter and gain their support, but remember friends will invariably, by definition, take your side so you need professional advice.

- Seek help, talk to a friend, approach a harassment advisor, speak to your manager (where they are not the bully) or speak to your trade union. Remember that the main aim of all good harassment procedures is to improve the working environment and ensure that harassment stops.

- As you work through the procedure you will need to have courage in approaching the bully. Utilise the support you have, and insist that the bullying stops. Be clear about the nature of the offensive behaviours and how you want to be treated. If the behaviours continue then return to your advisors and consider your next steps in line with your organisation's procedures.

- Objecting to workplace bullying is not easy, it takes courage and persistence. This is also true where you are supporting a colleague who complains to you that they have been or are being bullied. Use your knowledge of workplace bullying and your organisation's procedures to support and assist them. In some cases they may be mistaken, but treat their complaint seriously and supportively. Encourage them to take advice from appropriate quarters, and with support to insist that the bullying stops. In extreme cases you may need to support your colleague in reporting matters to the police where a criminal offence has taken place.

Important note: here I've concentrated on the 'victim' of the bullying; however, being a witness to bullying can be equally stressful. Observing bullying acts can mean that you experience the same level of violence, intimidation, disrespect and unfairness in the workplace. Indeed, in some cases the signal towards observers may be even more powerful than that to the 'victim'.

Therefore if you observe workplace bullying you need to act. Make it clear to the bully that they are corrupting your work environment and that this is unacceptable. This takes courage, but bullying prospers where workers neglect to object.

Related legislation

Various pieces of legislation on the statute book in the UK appear, superficially, to relate to the problem of harassment at work. Are these useful, and how can this legislation assist an individual who may experience harassment at work?

A list of related legislation may be presented as follows:

- The Protection of Harassment Act (1997)
- The Offences Against the Person Act (1998)
- The Sexual Offences Act (2003)
- The Health and Safety at Work Act (1974)
- The Disability Discrimination Act (1995)
- The Employment Rights Act (1996)
- The Employment Equality (Sex Discrimination) Act (2005)
- The Race Relations (Amendment) Act (2000)

It is worth considering these in turn in order to evaluate their relevance and usefulness in respect of workplace bullying.

The Protection of Harassment Act (1997)

Superficially this title could infer that this legislation is highly relevant. Actually, this legislation is specifically about 'stalking' and would be difficult to apply in a general sense in the workplace. This legislation would only apply where an individual has committed a stalking act. However, it may be worthwhile taking legal advice where harassment takes the form of physical or cyber-stalking.

The Offences Against the Person Act (1998)

This includes criminal offences against the person, including assault and causing injury. Bullying at work may include physical injury and assault, and if this occurs it constitutes a criminal act. Victims of assault would need to involve the police.

The Sexual Offences Act (2003)

This revises the law related to sexual offences such as rape, sexual assault and other offences and deals specifically with aspects of 'consent'. Thus, where bullying at work includes a sexual assault, the criminal law is again involved. 'Touching' of a sexual nature would certainly mean that the victim could make a complaint to the police.

The Health and Safety at Work Act (1974)

In many ways this is probably the most useful piece of legislation for protecting employees from bullying at work. Employers and individual managers have a 'duty of care' to ensure a safe working environment, which includes protection related to psychological health. Under Section 2, employers have a general duty to ensure the health, safety and welfare at work of all their employees. This responsibility for health includes mental health.

Bullying at work may lead to mild or profound effects on mental health and wellbeing, and therefore employees and their trade unions can argue for protection from bullying at work using this legislation. Risk assessments should be requested where bullying at work is evident. It is always best to use any reference to health and safety issues in conjunction with using your organisation's harassment or bullying policy.

The Disability Discrimination Act (1995), The Employment Rights Act (1996), The Employment Equality (Sex Discrimination) Act (2005) and The Race Relations (Amendment) Act (2000)

These can be useful in setting the context and arguing individual cases where they present potential breaches of these pieces of legislation. If you are concerned get advice from a trade union or a solicitor. From 1 October 2005, the Employment Equality (Sex Discrimination) Regulations 2005 came into force. These changes include a new definition of harassment which includes both sex-related and sexual harassment. This legal change should provide a basis for challenging sexual harassment in the workplace.

Note concerning using legislation: please note that these distinctions are made based upon my experience as a harassment advisor and trade union caseworker. I am not a lawyer; they may take a different view. In most cases the issue will not get to court anyway, the essential element is the way in which reference to legal rights and responsibilities may alleviate the bullying problem.

Remember: your primary aim should be to stop the bullying.

As an aim this is always better than 'get revenge' or 'punish the bully'.

Moving towards a resolution that stops the bullying and restores respect and dignity at work is a very different aim; having this as your aim will positively affect your approach to the situation and the responses of other people, including the bully, managers who may support your actions, colleagues, etc.

Conclusion – and your action plan

In conclusion, we have examined the organisational context of workplace bullying and how research indicates that low job satisfaction and high role conflict and role ambiguity appear to co-exist with high incidence of bullying. We have also considered the various behaviours that can constitute workplace bullying.

In examining your responses to workplace bullying, as managers and as members of staff, you have considered whether bullying occurs in your workplace and how you can respond. We have examined how the law affects our responses to various kinds of workplace bullying.

In order to benefit from your consideration of workplace bullying, consider the following action plan:

1   having established your awareness of workplace bullying, resolve to maintain this by periodically reviewing this material
2   talk to colleagues about workplace bullying; these practices thrive where workers are afraid to talk openly

3 talk to your line manager about workplace bullying, and find a copy of your organisation's policy and/or procedure

4 try and get your manager to agree to some discussion about workplace bullying at a team meeting. Consider: how would we deal with this if it occurred here? What is the organisation's policy? Do we have a procedure? Do we have harassment advisors?

Finally, workplace environments can be supportive and encouraging. Where there is mutual respect and where co-workers deal with each other in a manner that maintains the dignity of all individuals, work is rewarding, fulfilling and enriching.

References

1 Adams A. *Bullying at Work – how to confront and overcome it*. London: Virago Press; 1992.

2 Adams A. *Bullying at Work*. London: Virago; 1996.

3 Field T. *Bully in Sight*. Wantage, Oxfordshire: Success Unlimited; 1996.

4 Randall P. *Adult Bullying: perpetrators and victims*. London: Routledge; 1997.

5 Einarsen S and Skogstad A. Bullying at work: epidemiological findings in public and private organisations. *European Journal of Work and Organisational Psychology*. 1996;5:185–201.

6 Einarsen S, Raknes BI and Matthiesen SB. Bullying and harassment at work and their relationship to work environment quality: an exploratory study. *European Work and Organizational Psychologist*. 1994;4:381–401.

7 Brodsky CM. *The Harassed Worker*. Toronto: Lexington Books; 1976.

8 Olweus D. *Aggression in the Schools: bullies and whipping boys*. Washington DC: Hemisphere (Wiley); 1978.

9 Felson RB. 'Kick 'em, when they're down': explanations of the relationships between stress and interpersonal aggression and violence. *The Sociological Quarterly*. 1992;33:1–16.

10 Einarsen S (ed.). *Bullying and Harassment at Work: epidemiological and psychosocial aspects*. Bergen: University of Bergen; 1996.

11 Leymann H. Mobbing and psychological terror at workplaces. *Violence and Victims*. 1990;5:119–26.

12 Kahn RL, Wolfe DM, Quinn RP and Snoek JD. *Organisational Stress: studies in role conflict and ambiguity*. New York: Wiley; 1982.

13 Kahn H and Cooper CL. *Stress in the Dealing Room*. London: Routledge; 1993.

14 French JRP and Caplan RD. Psychosocial factors in coronary heart disease. *Industrial Medicine*. 1970;39:383–97.

15 Shiron A, Eden D, Silbberwasser S and Kellerman JJ. Job stress and risk factors in coronary heart disease among occupational categories in Kibbutzim. *Social Science and Medicine*. 1973; 7:875–92.

16 Kahn RL. Role conflict and ambiguity in organisations. In: Mattesson MT and Ivancevich JM (eds). *Management and Organisational Behaviour Classics*. Homewood, Illinois: Irwin; 1989.

17 Einarsen S and Raknes BI. Harassment in the workplace and the victimization of men. In: Einarsen S (ed.). *Bullying and Harassment at Work: epidemiological and psychosocial aspects*. Bergen: University of Bergen; 1996.

18 Szilagyi AD, Sims HP and Keller RT. Role dynamics, locus of control and employee attitudes and behaviour. *Academy of Management Journal*. 1976;19:259–76.

19 Bedeian AG and Armenakis AA. A path-analytic study of the consequences of role conflict and ambiguity. *Academy of Management Journal*. 1981;24:417–24.

20 Leymann H. *Vuxenmobbning – om Psykist vold I Arbetslivet* [Adult bullying: psychological terror at work]. Lund, Sweden: Studentlitteratur; 1976.

21 O'Brien GE, Dowling P and Kobanoff B. *Work, Health and Leisure* (report No.1). Adelaide, Australia: Department of Social Security, Flinders University; 1977.

22 Marek J, Tangenes B and Hellesoy OH. *Organisational and Social Aspects of Jobs in Work Environment Statfjord Field. Work environment, health and safety on a North Sea oil platform*. Oslo, Norway: Universitetsforlaget AS; 1984: pp. 198–229.

23 Rizzo J, House RJ and Lirtsman SI. Role conflict and ambiguity in complex organisations. *Administrative Science Quarterly*. 1970;15:150–63.

Chapter 3

Organisational accounts of bullying: an interactive approach

Malcolm Lewis

The information in this chapter is based in part on my research of nurse managers' and nurses' constructions of bullying in the NHS.[1] The chapter is based around a number of accounts of bullying within the NHS and is applicable to all healthcare professionals. While bullying is a complex process, by looking at the scenarios you will be able to better understand bullying mechanisms from a number of angles. You will see how:

- bullying activity emerges
- bullying can influence professional actions
- the NHS as an organisation may be dealing with it
- victims of bullying may be at a disadvantage when attempting to gain redress for such acts.

The chapter focuses upon subjective experiences of healthcare professionals as they attempt to deal with bullying. You will gain an understanding of bullying not simply as a psychological or deviant process, but as one in which bullies and victims are actively constructing the bullying situation in the NHS.

Bullying emergence

The emergence of bullying behaviour is a complex and detailed process. Bullying is identified here as a learned process which is very much organisationally mediated in the NHS. I wish to offer an alternative account to those theorists who see the bully as having certain personality traits. I think that what are essentially seen as 'personality differences' arise from beliefs and the values inherent in the NHS workplace.

As we have seen in the previous two chapters, various theorists have speculated as to why an individual may bully, or what may act as a trigger to lead to bullying.[2–4] Trying to explain why people bully has presented considerable problems for researchers, and similarly definitions of bullying are still being debated.[5] A central theme has been one of intentionality, i.e. does an individual intend to, or actively seek to bully another person? There seems to be evidence enough to indicate that individuals do bully with intent and with malice, and that they may also develop 'serial' bullying behaviours.[6]

The serial bully is the individual who continues bullying over a period of time by focusing on a variety of victims in the workplace, and this is not an uncommon situation in healthcare. These bullies tend to follow a classic bullying career; they are often well known, but little complained about. Activities may be associated closely with clique (favoured group) behaviour. It is in such close-knit communities that bullying may flourish, and in particular serial bullying behaviour develops. This is not universally the case, but it would appear to be common enough.

Here is an example from Sharon, a staff nurse in intensive care who is being bullied by the senior sister; she gives an example of her situation:

> The clique of people ... as time unfolded ... and I got friendly with the nicer people they would actually tell me of their experience ... I mean these were women in their 40s and 50s who were now upper grades. They'd come in as D grades and been in the same position as I was but worked through it. One was a sister who'd been I'd say intimidated, but refused to respond really. An E grade who had been demoted due to this same person, and also an F grade that had a lot of trauma in her personal life. They also experienced bullying from this particular woman. All three of them had come to me, because I think [of] things they'd seen. Things happening in the unit they knew that I was being, erm, I say bullied.

She indicates how bullying can continue and can move from staff member to staff member, all of them being bullied by the same person. Sharon then comments upon the bully's activities and the timeframe:

> Erm, they'd ignored it all for too long ... 15 years this woman had been working there, and 15 years of bullying really. A girl prior to me, three years before I came had actually taken her to a disciplinary hearing. She had a file with the harassment officer.

In Sharon's view:

- very little was seen to be done about the bullying
- specific individuals became targets over long time periods, shifting from staff member to staff member
- it is an example of serial bullying.

Einarsen has regarded the issue of bullying as a unified phenomenon, in that bullying is an ongoing activity – it has a 'career' nature and can be seen as a process where definitions are constantly being redefined by the bully and victim.[6] This 'career' can be seen in the above scenario, and Sharon's view identifies the characteristics of a career – it is intentional and organised and occurs over a long period of time with numerous victims.

Bullying and personality

The notion of bullies being 'weak' individuals is a common theme in the literature.[7] There are similarities in arguments with victims also being seen as weak, or being unable to 'stand up to the bully'. Indeed, in my study, victims do not come across as weak, but often as clear thinking and proactive individuals faced with a bullying problem; and this is probably the case with the majority of victims who are healthcare professionals. Bullies themselves may be far from weak when we consider the degree of manipulation and sophistication associated with many bullying events.

We are, however, at a distinct disadvantage in the study of bullies, as knowledge of them is derived mainly from their victims, who may have their own particular definitions of the bullying.[8] Data on bullies remain controversial. Peter Randall is one of the major proponents of the argument that bullies demonstrate weaknesses and they possess inadequate personalities.[2] Other studies have contrastingly seen bullies as self-confident, but nevertheless impulsive in their nature.[9] Field is broadly in agreement with Randall, but believes that bullies have low self-esteem, which is related in part to a fear of their shortcomings being revealed.[7]

According to such approaches, bullies discover in childhood the appropriate behaviours to support bullying. Randall has contended that psychodynamic counselling often reveals such patterns or traits in behaviour.[2] Quite often though, such traits are looked for *after* episodes of bullying. It is quite common that many healthcare professionals are told they have a 'personality clash' with the bully and need counselling, which rarely gets to the bottom of the bullying.

We should remember also that such bullying personality profiles do not fit comfortably with the role of healthcare professionals, in that many healthcare professionals do not fit the pattern of being psychologically weak, particularly considering the complex roles they often undertake.

Personality traits aside, intentionality does appear to be a common characteristic of bullying. Here is Steve (a nurse manager in psychiatry) clearly indicating in this example that much bullying may be intentional:

> I feel bullying is more about intent than accident. I think, erm, maybe the distinction between bullying and not bullying apart from the perception of the person who feels they are being bullied. I think is about intent, to a large element ... I suppose you can be unfair without the intent but this is, you actually choose to abuse someone don't you? You choose to exclude them, you choose to do things, and these are actions rather than inaction. Well, inaction can be just as bad, you know, choosing not to do something, but again it's proper choice, and it's an active thing isn't it ... even if it's inaction it's active.

Here then, Steve perceives a number of issues relevant to our discussion:

- bullying would appear not to be accidental; the bully is aware
- individual perception is important (i.e. how we label bullying)
- there is an option to do something, or to do nothing in relation to the bullying – we have a choice.

Brim sees personality traits of the bully developing only in terms of perceived attitudes of an individual as they are defined and expressed in the social context.[10] In the case of healthcare professionals this is influenced to a large degree by the workplace and in interactions with work colleagues. In such a situation the dynamics of any bullying behaviours become complicated. Leymann has focused on the work environment, and reminds us of differing bullying behaviours exhibited in differing organisational contexts (despite the existence of certain core bullying actions).[11] He sees bullying as being a dynamic and transactional process over time, and that bullies and victims are not passive, but active in their decisions and acts.

Here is Jenny, an experienced practice nurse, focusing upon bullying around managers. She sees healthcare managers as possibly projecting their inadequacies on staff, which may or may not denote an intention to bully:

> Managers are trying to mould behaviour, quite creative ... the manager's background and history influences them covering their back.

Managers then may be:

- covering their backs
- creative in bullying
- influenced by history and background.

How does this equate with bullying? In Jenny's view the bully (in this case, managers) may be highly manipulative, and bullying may be part of this manipulation. Being creative does not seem to equate with weakness, but she is also quite clear that they have learned such 'tricks of the trade' from experience and interaction in the workplace. A major finding in my study was the identification of nursing managers being both the perpetrators and victims of bullying at the same time, and it would appear that this trend is repeated throughout the healthcare workforce.

How are bullying acts emerging?

Bullying emerges as health professionals become influenced by the culture in any particular group. Waller indicates that many people interacting in group life have mapped out and influenced, pre-existing definitions of the situation.[12] Bullies continually define and redefine situations in respect of bullying. Clearly it seems people are influenced by group norms but while we may all have the potential for bullying behaviour, it does not always emerge. Here are the views of Pauline, who works in organ retention and control and has some 34 years of nursing experience:

> Bullying occurs in times of transition, where the status quo is changing.
> It provides an opportunity for the bully to come into place.

Pauline's comment may give us further clues to what may be occurring in healthcare bullying situations. It may also support the notion of the bully as a competent social actor:

- the bully may be an opportunist (which in itself indicates a degree of foresight and knowledge)
- change is perceived by many to be traumatic; it may, as Pauline indicates, provide an 'opportunity for the bully to come into place'
- such instability in the healthcare work environment may be contributing to the perceived rise in bullying activity. However, some behaviours may be defined as bullying which in less unstable situations may not be.

The act of bullying being defined in different ways and by different groups in healthcare in itself gives rise to conflict. In such a scenario, the social life of the hospital or healthcare environment can be seen as a mass of such situations and definitions. In this sense it can act as an agent of social control in that it transmits to its workers attitudes of those 'gone before'.

If the bully has the support of a clique and is able to influence them, a situation develops in which the bullying may be allowed to continue and it is not questioned. Indeed, staff may do little to stop it, even when they become aware of it and where it may seriously damage career prospects.

In the bully's interaction with others they learn how to use appropriate behaviour to justify the bullying (although they will not call it that). Such manipulation by bullies remains complex, which is precisely what contributes to confusion in defining bullying and the difficulty of obtaining adequate redress for many victims of bullying.

The bully as a manipulator

Here is Diana, a medical nursing manager, discussing the difficulties of dealing with the bully, mainly because of the confusion surrounding definitions, but also because the bully can be manipulative and act in appropriate ways to justify or manipulate their actions. In this case she is discussing the difficulty unions have, and why they may be supportive of the bully:

> I think that's the sort of thing where unions sort of jump on it, you know, that they're not treating the bully properly. Erm, never mind the victim, they're, it's almost as if the union stands up for the bully, you know and it's ... sometimes I do think that the bully almost turns ... turns themselves into the victim.

Again, Diana's account raises a number of points:

- the bully is acting with forethought
- they are seen to manipulate situations (in influencing union opinion)
- such is the fluency of this action that they may be able to turn the situation to their advantage and see themselves as victims.

Burke reminds us that when we bully, we are performing for an audience.[14] In cases of cliques and of group bullying, the bully has a ready-made audience to play to, and such may be the strength of the performance by the bully that rarely are their actions challenged or even regarded as bullying by colleagues. Such then may be the manipulative acumen of the bully that a victim may remain unsure if they are being bullied. This leads us into a possible explanation for the difficulties in establishing what is bullying behaviour, frequently until very late in the process.

I have already indicated how bullies may be particularly manipulative in their actions. Indeed, recent thinking by Raynor, Hinton, and Petri is showing some concern about seeing the bully as either 'incompetent' or 'deficient'.[14–16] Bullies would not be able to bully at all unless they devised definitions of their specific situations, inferring they are competent. If we can accept this, then intentional bullying demonstrates awareness of what they are doing from the outset. In cases where unwitting bullying is happening (where an individual may be accused of bullying but is not aware that what they are doing is bullying behaviour), once the individual is made aware of the consequences of his/her actions, the bullying should stop.

Consider now this quote from Jenny, a practice nurse bullied by her colleague (a doctor), whose discussion turns to why bullies act as they do. She is quite clear as to what the bully is doing:

> Bullying is manipulative and calculating behaviour ... I think for their own ends really, they are trying to get what they want irrespective of who they are bullying, and the substance, and if they can't find behaviour that, that requires, erm, changing, then they make it up.

Jenny is very clear about how she sees the bully, and how they focus on behaviour. Being focused to get what they want and being manipulative in getting it requires a fair degree of insight and possible planning. In Jenny's situation the bully is seen as being reflective, and therefore able to understand the differences between what constitutes accidental and intended behaviour.

She indicates a recurring theme:

- bullies may not be the weak individuals some researchers claim
- manipulating behaviour may be seen as a reasonable tactic if it is to get what they want
- such activity again requires reflection and planning.

Sutton *et al.*, in a critique of the view that the bully is somehow deficient, present an alternative view to the common 'oafish' stereotype of the bully.[17] The degree of social manipulation used by bullies then may be highly sophisticated. The use of indirect and covert bullying methods such as social isolation, exclusion tactics, setting up to fail, etc. requires knowledge by the bully of the social infrastructure of the healthcare environment.

This is perhaps more clearly seen in the activities of serial bullying, where there may be continuation, fluency, and an increasing sophistication of bullying techniques over time. Sophistication in bullying tends to increase as one gets older, and may manifest in increasingly novel ways of avoiding detection (with experience).

The problem of bullying awareness

Bullying events are often complex and take place often over extended timeframes. Great variability has been identified in how awareness of bullying develops in both bullies and their victims. In my research I made a detailed re-examination of Glaser and Strauss's work on awareness contexts and its application to bullying events.[18] Although their original work is focused upon awareness of the dying patient in hospital, the essential features associated with Glaser and Strauss's original concepts of awareness can be seen when examining bullying.

Such an approach allows one to analyse the 'passage' of the individual's awareness of a significant event, in this instance, the bullying. This allows bullying acts to be examined over time, as often in healthcare bullying is found to be a long and complicated event. Often healthcare workers do not label bullying, and situations may improve or deteriorate, with change in working and organisational factors leading to a slow or sometimes rapid awareness of bullying events. Many victims are often confused as to when events first began.

Timescales and pretence

It is not unusual for victims to report problems over two- to three-year periods or longer, with durations of 6–12 months being common. As we have already seen, bullies can often manipulate the situation to their advantage, and the bully may be highly skilled in the manipulation of organisational use of rules and procedures, which can cover their actions under a cloak of legitimacy, i.e. demonstrate a state of pretence.

This is exacerbated as there are often shifting alliances, suspicion and denials. Contexts become rapidly unstable in bullying, with high levels of distrust and deceit, which ultimately complicates both its identification and resolution in organisations. Quite simply then, at what stage of the process do healthcare workers know they are being bullied? This is not such a straightforward question. Here is a typical quote from Pauline, a nurse in the community of many years' experience being bullied by her manager:

> I've learned a tremendous amount about myself. It's still not resolved. Well it was on reflection really. Yeah, but it's happened to me before, I realise now, but I didn't identify it three years ago as bullying.

Many accounts of bullying reveal the issue of gradual awareness and late definition of the term bullying. Awareness is rarely an instantaneous situation. Again this is demonstrated in the comments of Celia, a nurse manager in obstetrics and gynaecology who was bullied by her line manager:

> I don't suppose I ever thought it was bullying at the time. I just felt I was, well I was sent to Coventry. Looking back now with experience yes, it was bullying. The other staff only realised it was bullying 18 months down the line.

Issues here include:

- bullying not being called bullying
- abusive events almost seen as normal, i.e. being sent to Coventry
- perceived lack of awareness of other staff
- awareness developing over extended timeframes.

While pretence is a favourable situation for the determined bully at any time in the bullying event, a third party may alert either the bully or the victim to what may be 'going on'.

This is seen in Celia's previous account, in which staff eventually realised what was happening. This is not always the case as staff may be reluctant to come forward, as they fear becoming victims themselves and do not want 'to rock the boat'.

Emerson and Messinger have described how the awareness of a problem for an individual may develop slowly, from having vague feelings of there being 'something wrong', and on thinking about them, their beginning to be revealed as a problem.[19] They also indicate the cyclic nature of problematic events, i.e. that problems may be resolved (or appear to be), or that something works for a time, only to be partly resolved, or resolved only in the eyes of one party. This may be seen where the bully may concede to the views of the victim, or aim for reconciliation. In such situations the complaints by the victim may be 'dropped', or the problem redefined, and potential damage to the bully limited, only allowing the situation to go unresolved.

We can now summarise some important points:

- many healthcare workers are still unaware of issues surrounding bullying and its definition
- awareness of bullying may often be brought about by a trigger or significant event that raises awareness, or by colleagues
- the possibility of pretence in bullying is great. Bullies may feign ignorance, put the blame on the victim and carefully manage situations to their advantage
- such actions by the bully are particularly covert in healthcare organisations, and tend to increase with the age and experience of the bully
- serial bullying must be considered. This is common when complaints and history are looked at in healthcare settings
- the longer a state of pretence or manipulation continues, the more the danger of disclosure increases, and states of suspicion and eventual open awareness will develop. Third parties, e.g. colleagues, may get increasingly suspicious that 'all is not right'.

Effects of trigger events

Trigger events may be revealed unwittingly by others, or may be more direct either to confirm suspicion or confirm bullying is happening. The effects of triggers can be devastating for the bully as they are a cause of exposure. One way a trigger may be initiated is with an 'angry outburst' on the part of the bully which exposes behaviour that has usually been progressing for some time. Here is an example of just such an outburst, which is all too public. In this case it involved a nurse manager in paediatrics. Yvonne recalls an incident in theatre when she was identifying ongoing bullying by a consultant:

> I wouldn't take a child back from theatre because it was an intensive care patient and it was a high-dependency unit, and I flatly refused to. The consultant came in and shouted at me, and I told him to wait and I rang my general manager because I couldn't get hold of the ward manager ... I'd just had enough at that point. I actually took a month's unpaid leave and went travelling and came back. The same was happening to all staff, but they were getting on with it, been pressured to take patients they couldn't cope with.

Notice here again:

- a reluctance of staff to complain
- the initiation of the trigger in an angry outburst
- the action of the victim in interpreting the situation and removing themselves from the influence of such bullying.

Again the label 'bully' is infrequently used by health professionals, but it tends to be used with hindsight and retrospectively.

This can also be seen in the experiences of Jenny, an experienced practice nurse being bullied by her general practitioner (GP) boss. She raised a number of issues over a considerable time period, regarding how she had to reorganise her work while being subjected to bullying. In this instance it included criticism of her organisation, her dealing with patient issues and appointments, and her clinical skills. Eventually she labels the actions of her GP boss as bullying. The incident she recounts some time into the episode indicates she is clearly aware that something is wrong when her work is criticised. She is accused of making mistakes, and she concentrates a great deal on maintaining her professional standards, and feels initially that it must be some fault of hers for failing to maintain such standards. This is at a time when her work is focused on major change. She says:

> This, right, the start of the National Service Frameworks and we had a new partner taken on, erm, seemed a nice chap, a Lebanese guy, erm, what they did they printed out, to get your National Service Framework Heart Disease Register, they printed out this thing on computer and they realised I'd been making mistakes. I felt really, I just wanted to get out and run out, I felt threatened.

What follows from this is the involvement of the new doctor in a meeting along with the senior GP whom she eventually labelled as the bully. She was summoned to a meeting with no prior warning and reprimanded over her 'mistakes'. Even though this is not the first incident in the process Jenny generally felt nothing was wrong. She continues:

> No, because I said to them tell me if there is something you don't like me doing, let me know ... no one had said a sausage.

A significant (trigger) event occurs at the end of a further meeting regarding her 'progress' in the practice. She continues:

> So, I, I mean he said, erm, you will come back on Monday morning for a disciplinary hearing, and I was shown off the premises [laughs] by his administrative assistant. I got my coat and my bag and I left in tears.

She recounts in her interview how she perceives she is being treated unfairly. She was shocked by the proceedings and begins to consider the possibility that she is being bullied:

> Well, that particular incident I felt very threatened, so, I presume I would call it bullying.

Ultimately, this results in Jenny arriving home in tears and her husband contacting the surgery in a state of anger to inform them she will not be returning on the Monday for a disciplinary hearing. Jenny's events are not untypical, and illustrate the slow emergence of the bully label.

It is in situations like this that one may wonder why action has not taken place earlier, and why such acts are allowed to continue. The possibility may arise of a situation in which bullying is seen as the norm in a particular working situation and environment, and is defined as such by participants. O'Connell et al. have suggested that in situations of repeated and long-term exposure to bullying, a state of sensitisation may occur, not only in the perception of the victim but also on the part of any who observe such acts.[20] In such situations it may appear as the norm to the social group and spread throughout it. In particular, the victim may fail to get support and help early in the event, and isolation increases, particularly in their ability to get help from the bully's 'helpers'.

Many managers, then, either identify that they themselves are not aware of bullying, that they could not identify others calling it that, or that while they are still not aware they may identify a suspicious state in the victim. Here is Steve's view. What is particularly problematic in the managerial situation is that while managers are being accused of being the bully, many of them in turn are bullied by senior managers:

> Mmm [pause] I don't know from my point of view. I didn't perceive it as bullying, that I was being bullied until I did some studying into bullying. Ermm, and maybe that's just about terminology really.

In Steve's case we see:

- difficulty with terminology, and an admission of not being aware of bullying
- not being aware that he was bullying, as indicated in the following statement:
  Well, I felt you bullied me ... bullied me into taking more people, and I said 'bullied?' ... because it was the actual ... she used the word bullying, she said, well, maybe not bullied ... but maybe pressured to take on more people.

Note here how:

- the subordinate turns the tables on the manager with an accusation of bullying, indicating she is also a victim although she downgrades the statement
- Steve, while surprised, now becomes suspicious of bullying – a trigger has occurred.

Downgrading from the term 'bullying' is also seen in Yvonne's comments, a paediatric nurse manager:

> I don't know if I would term it bullying, because bullying to me is what kids do to each other. That's just my impression, and, I was bullied at school ... when somebody is unkind to somebody else ... I've had managers shout at me because something was going wrong somewhere else ... I wouldn't say that was bullying.

Again there is the reluctance to admit to the word 'bully', and often a confirmation that there is nothing abnormal going on, and no need to complain. However, with their increased experience, and with the knowledge of their superior position, the bullying manager may take on a degree of confidence and authority that creates a growing state of awareness in the victim, and a growing sense of control and power in the bully. Such is the ability to manipulate that while bullying actions can bring about suspicion, it is often a time of doubt and uncertainty in the victim. It is also a stage of manipulation where the bully can begin a process of 'blame reversal'.

Again managers may admit to the use of bullying quite openly as a tactic. Anna, a medical nurse manager, justifies the use of coercive tactics but angles her actions from the need to maintain staff 'competencies'. She admits she and other managers have used this tactic; she says:

> Bullying in nursing is not seen as bullying, people look at competencies. And they use it as that angle ... You are not coming up to competency, or

you are not coming up to your role. Therefore I want you to come up to your role ... nurses can be blinkered. They don't always see the other person's point of view.

As we have already seen, clashes of differing personality is another issue and it is raised by many managers and NHS trusts in dealing with bullying behaviour. It is a mechanism frequently employed at an organisational level once awareness of bullying has been established. Invariably the victim is seen as having a clash of interests with the bully, and if action is taken the victim is frequently moved or offered counselling to help them adjust.

One of the victims in my study, despite winning many thousands of pounds at a tribunal against her trust for bullying, is indignant that both the bully and trust deny anything is wrong, and say that it was all a 'personality clash'. Often victims are not believed, and again have an uphill struggle on their hands and feel they are up against the system, with bullies fighting their own corners to not 'rock the boat'. Furthermore, managers who are bullies may consider they are also more powerful and can impose sanctions on victims who try to expose their activities. Likewise age may be a factor, as the older manager has usually been in the healthcare situation longer, and may be more conversant with policy and procedure and how to manipulate these to their own ends.

In particular, serial bullies are also more prone to exposure due to the very nature and timing of their activities, and the fact the bully may have multiple victims at the same time. In all such situations the exposure risk increases, as does the need to hide the activities. The bully may help perpetuate this state in a number of ways:

- general bullying tactics, e.g. in particular isolation and undermining of victim confidence
- being aware that there is lack of knowledge about recognising bullying for what it is
- conflicts being seen as 'normal' and part of the everyday need to maintain standards and get work done
- staff fears, anxieties and insecurities, both in supporting victims and in wanting to avoid such conflict for themselves.

Suspicion of bullying therefore remains problematic and may be associated with:

- bullying taking place over extended timeframes, increasing the possibility of exposure
- perceptions of healthcare workers in how organisations handle events (issues of fairness, parity, etc.)
- multiple, perceived bullying events.

The issue as to when one becomes suspicious of bullying may also be influenced by a number of other factors. In research on nursing it has been observed that in verbal abuse of nurses, abusive nurses are often distinguished in terms of their position.[21] Indeed, the higher the status of bullies in the eyes of the victims, the more their actions may be seen as meaningful and alternatively these actions are less likely to arouse suspicion. Interestingly, the traditional hierarchical status of nursing may itself act as a mechanism to reduce the complaints of bullying by nurses. It may be perceived that in such situations the behaviour of higher status nurses may be difficult to control, not least due to the fact that they have more organisational power and access to resources, and also that the bully may follow through on any threats they make.

It may be seen that to complain may have little impact on events; it also brings into question the efficacy of organisational systems and structures which may be organised in such a way as to allow this to happen in the first place. Such conditions can actually favour the actions of the bully, and can support situations of pretence. Often in the experiences of these nurses there is a feeling of almost total failure if they have to admit to needing help – a form of weakness in an otherwise 'stoic professional'.

This effect is not unusual in bullying in general, as many bullied individuals are made to feel such problems are all of their own making and that they are powerless to do anything about it. It is such events that support notions of victims having 'inadequate personalities'. This may be one reason why the realisation of being bullied is, on the whole, a slow and painful process. It seems almost incredible in some situations that such destructive events are allowed to continue. In such bad situations, denial may be a way for the victim to stay in a bad situation from which they cannot escape. For instance, just leaving one's job, or even being able to move from a job or area are not viable options for many who may have family or other commitments.

Phillip, a surgical nursing manager, is aware of this and indicates that suspicion may be present in both parties, but failure to act may be due to fear. Indeed in such situations a condition of 'mutual pretence' awareness may develop to maintain a sense of status quo. He continues:

> We can't stop NHS bullying if we first don't accept that it exists. People need to stand up and say it is happening, but are afraid of retribution.

This statement reflects on wider conditions in the NHS as an organisation and its ability to apply possible censure and retribution if such events are reported. There is both a fear and a reluctance to acknowledge and communicate effectively about bullying and it is therefore not surprising little is known about it.

Open awareness of bullying

Even where the bully has been openly accused of bullying they may still show pretence and either deliberately deny bullying or genuinely not acknowledge bullying at all. Another problem here is that in open awareness, bringing bullying literally 'out into the open' brings the possibility of confrontation, and exposes the fact that something should be done about it. This is not a straightforward issue, as both parties may want different outcomes, which may not result in any resolution.

Differences in perceptions and rights and responsibilities may be asserted or contested as the situation becomes publicised.[19] The situation may be strongly contested, often with the bully seeing the victim as the source of trouble. One trigger repeatedly identified with bullying is organisational change and changes in work practices. When Mary talks about the start of her bullying episode, she relates it to the emergence and demands of GP fundholding:

> I'd come back from maternity leave having had my little boy; I'd been working in the practice for a few months and we were told that GP fundholding was beginning to come into force ... As a result of that it

meant we had two weeks' notice to find other jobs within the trust but fortunately we were helped by our director of nursing and nurse manager. We were all split up and put into different teams. I myself was put in one area, and this is where the problem started. I felt I was sent to an area I could not handle.

In this instance Mary had been moved from one work context to another, and felt that this contributed to her problems; she felt that she was placed in a situation that set her up to fail. She recounts later how the bullying continues by another member of staff (a sister) as she continues to work on the district. Even after a fairly prolonged episode, and specific trigger events, Mary only uses the word bullying late on in her account, but remains clear about what was happening to her.

Managerial control and lack of support

Next we hear from Sandra, an occupational health nurse who found her company was far from supportive. She identified bullying from her healthcare manager, who was not a nurse but a health and safety expert and had been brought in new to the post and was making changes in her occupational health unit. Sandra ultimately gets support from both the occupational physician and another colleague; however, the manager does not see his actions as bullying but rather as necessary managerial action to run the unit efficiently.

When Sandra reports the problem to a more senior manager who informs the bully, she continues to be ostracised. Sandra also raises questions of patient confidentiality and professional concerns. She felt that her practice was being compromised. When asked why she identified this as bullying she says:

> Why was it bullying? ... Because of standing, having to explain what you were doing, you weren't allowed to do your job properly if you, you know, didn't go in the morning you were reprimanded and reported ... we couldn't see to our patients.

In this incident Sandra mentions that both herself and the other nursing staff were made to form a semicircle on coming into work in the morning and report on their intended day's activities to the manager. She felt she was increasingly controlled and threatened by the manager who also demanded access to patients' notes. She continues:

> I felt threatened because nothing was being done about confidentiality. I thought I was going to be struck off ... if the UKCC [United Kingdom Central Council] found out ... It got to the stage where he wanted to ... you know, I said in the end 'do you want to come in and sit with me while I see to my patients?'. This is how bad it was getting.

Here we see:

- increasing control, not just strong management
- threat
- interference with professional autonomy
- continued trauma for the victim.

There was never an admission of bullying from this manager, even when the situation was taken further and dealt with by senior management. Sandra accuses both her manager and senior management of not listening, and of giving minimal support even when the event was out in the open and a formal accusation of bullying was made.

In the following quote from Celia, there is an obvious reference to bullying behaviour, and an admission that it was a tactic she used on her staff. She assured me that staff would not call it that as work had to be done. She says:

> Well you know they deserve it because I need this work doing, and I've asked for this work to be done.

Hazel, a manager from surgery, also justifies bullying, but notes that staff may just complain if there are decisions made which they don't want to hear (so don't tell them, she advises), while the use of bullying as a word is discouraged:

> People can use power in different ways, and there is an option for managers to bully ... they can lay rumours to undermine. Senior managers may keep information back ... the nurse manager acts more to disadvantage staff, which is easier to cover up so as not to be found out.

And here is Tina, an obstetric manager, reflecting that managers know what is happening, but prefer to ignore issues, not wanting to blow the whistle but preferring just to go through the motions:

> It's fear of blowing the whistle ... you read in the press about what happens to staff who make complaints or identify problem areas, and you go through and nothing gets done, and that's still happening.

Here bullying is being openly justified by the healthcare manager.

The ability to confuse victims, or divert awareness from them being bullied (despite some managers openly seeing their actions as such) illustrates the devious nature of the phenomenon, and openly illustrates bullying tactics. Such situations are not confined only to healthcare. In a recent correspondence with Munday, I discussed this problem of deception with respect to his study of teacher bullying, and in the manipulation of formal disciplinary procedures to support bullying actions (K Munday, personal communication, 2004). Munday's work shows clear and obvious intent on the part of the bully, and is a classic example of redirecting attention towards victim blaming.

The desire to get work done, by whatever means possible, is again illustrated in the comments of Sheena, another nurse manager. If this involves intimidation and verbal abuse then this too is seen as a valid activity occasionally. Sheena here is fully aware of her actions, but prefers not to call this bullying. She uses such tactics, but again while the victims of such abuse are undoubtedly aware of being on the receiving end, they may not label it as bullying. She says:

> Maybe [it is] valid to comment on others depending upon what level you are at. Provided you get X, Y and Z done in time it doesn't matter how it's done if the person is still producing the work.

The need for getting work done is seen again as justification for such actions, and a notion that the more senior you are the more appropriate it may be to use such an option. Note how Diana is quite clear about bullying:

> One-to-one bullying happens to managers ... a *fait acompli*, and we do it to staff, it's just not effective managing.

There is an open admission to bullying, but it is often used and manipulated in such a way as to avoid its definition by the victim, and is justified by recourse to, in the main, getting a job done, even if it is seen as not effective managing. It is likewise passed down from the top to the more junior managers, who are also expected to perform.

Phillip's earlier comment reiterates that even in situations of mutual suspicion people may not admit to bullying:

> We can't stop NHS bullying if we first don't accept that it exists. People need to stand up and say it is happening, but are afraid of retribution.

Phillip gives clues as to what the situation may be in the wider organisation, and the climate of silence and fear that permeates the notion of bullying, which can easily allow a situation to both continue and develop with disastrous consequences for all concerned. One effect of such situations can be the bully's assertion of being a victim and portraying themselves as an injured party. An example of such action, where the bully begins to turn the tables to act as if injured, is seen in Yvonne's account of dealing with a bullying staff member. In such situations the bully is exposed, but still attempts to manipulate the context:

> No, no, she categorically denied she, erm, was in any way, shape or form like this [a bully]. Started crying in front of these two girls and said I had got her under too much pressure and expected too much of her. At which stage one of the staff nurses just laughed her head off almost hysterically, erm, she put it back at me. So I started to take things off her.

In this situation the manager relents, and removes some of the pressure of work from the bully, and the bully conditionally claims victim status. Indeed, she turns the situation around to blame the manager. A similar situation occurred in Yvonne's case when members of nursing staff identified the bully (a case of peer bullying on this occasion) causing problems in their paediatric unit. This group's awareness left the bully in no doubt she had been identified, and at that stage she changed her ways.

It is not unusual then to discover that bullies either soften or deny the problem of bullying once it is out in the open. Even though victims may show awareness, they may have difficulty in taking any organisational action. They may be too afraid, or others may try to change their view in not admitting that such actions are bullying. This last option may be more common than it appears in an organisation that has a reluctance to admit to bullying events, or even pretends they are not happening.

Box 3.1 Summary

- Bullying is considered by some at times 'appropriate if work needs to be done'.
- Staff 'need to work harder', as health organisations are increasingly reacting to change.
- Bullying is embedded in the act of 'management' (although it is not called that, but neither is it strong or effective management).
- Bullying is openly justified by some managers.
- Managers can manipulate situations, information, etc. as a tactic.
- Staff may not complain for fear of their position, career, etc.

Organisational issues: rhetoric, reality and negotiations

A central strand to my research is the impact of the work organisation as being a central focus in both the creation and sustainability of bullying behaviour in healthcare. The NHS is problematic due to its complexity and size. As Handy argues, organisations of such complexity represent myriad internal structures and working arrangements.[22] Raynor suggests that this complexity is in part arising from the NHS' organisational power profile and from a need to deal with a variety of professions and professional groups.[14] She advocates that such professional structures that exist within the NHS lead to different treatment being meted out to different groups – notably thus leading to permissible unequal treatment. This is evidenced by Frank who notes this type of activity. He says:

> If you consider everything from the Bristol Inquiry to the attitude of consultants within hospitals when challenged, the staff are blamed for making the challenge. So for example, if a surgeon throws a scalpel at a theatre nurse in a bad mood, and it's picking on her and she complains, it's still the culture whereby it wouldn't be the consultant that would become the focus of the problem.

Indeed, according to Mary such complaining may lead to further bullying. She comments when talking about a bullied nurse:

> The nurse is very brave at reporting unsafe practices ... because of this she had been subjected to bullying.

Such comments raise a number of issues that we should be concerned about:

- victims of bullying may well find it difficult to complain about events in healthcare settings
- there is a feeling by some that they may be victims and be bullied if they complain
- there is a perception of a 'them and us' situation and a culture of blame.

Most of the bullying identified here is intraprofessional. For a caring group such as nurses it brings into question their concern and support for fellow colleagues. Nurses are clearly not a homogenous professional group, even if surface impressions may give this appearance.[4,23] This in itself sets conditions likely to breed intraprofessional conflict. At the same time, such aspirations also set up conditions for interprofessional conflict, for instance between medicine, management, and other professional groups.

Whilst Davies suggests that nurses are striving towards liberation from traditional oppression,[25] another area of concern in bullying studies has been the relationship between bullying behaviour and gender. Previous work in this area is variable (although many managers identified as bullies are men), while this current research identifies no strong trends towards a gender bias. However, Yvonne, for instance, comments on the following:

> I've worked in predominantly women areas since I did my training, and I've never known a bigger bunch of people that backbite about each other in my life.

Yvonne is making a very general statement, but in respect of bullying it would appear that females are more prone to use covert bullying methods overall.

Intraprofessional conflicts become more focused when examining the emergence of conflicting groups in nursing, and the growth of healthcare specialists in all areas. This itself may be fertile ground for the development of cliques. Often such groups are perceived as more desirable and of higher status than other healthcare or nursing groups. Likewise the growth of professional associations, particularly within nursing, such as theatre nurses, oncology nurses, trauma nurses amongst others, may themselves form clique groups. Benson argues there are going to be inevitable strains and conflicts as the potential exists within organisational members to pursue their individual or group agendas.[26]

As already noted, nurses and managers in my research have all alluded both to the rapid pace of change in healthcare and to the stressful nature of the jobs they do. There is an obvious concern with such pressures and bullying events. Frank is quite clear on this:

> The concepts of, erm, doing stuff in your own time is a form of bullying; it's typical, and I think used a lot in the NHS. Expecting people to work longer hours as unpaid hours and using their own time ... I think that's organisational bullying.

Healthcare can be in itself a route to power.[27] Control of health agendas by government and civil servants, and the prominence of doctors and general managers and administrators in itself may reduce any sense of high self-esteem in healthcare workers. There may be considerable conflict in the healthcare role, considering the stresses healthcare workers encounter in working in formal organisations such as the NHS, whose values are likely to be different from those of their own professional agenda. This conflict is exacerbated when they are expected to meet often difficult and compelling demands from others' expectations – notably, and increasingly, those of general managers.[28]

On one level, the demands of acting professionally with patients at a functional level conflict with the requirements to relate often at personal levels with closeness and expression. This is further complicated by managerial agendas, often contrary to the notion of professional working, which emphasise effectiveness and efficiency measures that are often quite alien to many healthcare workers' thinking, or simply seen as a waste of time.[29] The particular problem of isolation has been identified as a key component in many healthcare workers' bullying experiences, where professional cohesion crumbles.

Assessing organisational adequacy in dealing with bullying

With the NHS being such a large and complex organisation, there are pockets of managerial excellence, as well as areas of less effective management in dealing with bullying episodes. However, many healthcare workers allude to the issue of keeping bullying quiet and low profile, of it being nebulous and hidden.

To be effective, policy and procedure should be visible, be appropriately applied and be capable of dealing with bullying episodes for the protection of all staff. However, a thorough review of organisational disciplinary and grievance procedures was a requirement of the Employment Act (2002), and there appears to be much flaunting of NHS 'zero tolerance' initiatives.[30] Keeping bullying secret is not a good communicative strategy, but it may be preferable to being seen as not coping or rocking the boat.

For any strategy to be effective, staff must be conversant and happy with its proposal and possible effects. In most instances strategies and established policies on harassment and on the use of grievance procedures fail to be effective in dealing with the problems of bullying, a major issue being that they must be directed through the manager/senior management – the possible bullying perpetrators.

Mary indicates her frustration at the way the organisation fails to deal with her bullying complaints, and in particular how the manager tried to limit her activities in this area. Organisationally this was done in a number of ways:

> We give no support to the bullied. We have a policy which nobody hopes will be used … I think it's a paper exercise. It's tick in the box. Trusts don't want the confrontation of it unless it gets into the union bracket. Unless it's actively pushed into their face and it has to be dealt with, they would rather people on the ground floor deal with it and it doesn't get through to the top so we can shield the board from these issues.

Often it is a common tactic to remove the victim from the situation when the real sources of the problem, the bully or bullies, remain in place. Such a tactic is perhaps a simpler option, but may send out an inappropriate message to others who frequently are only too aware of events, and thus contributes to continued organisational damage. More essentially, it totally fails to deal with the root of the bullying problem and thus becomes a major contributory factor to the continuance of serial bullying behaviour. The idea of a bullying situation being difficult to deal with does not act as an excuse for making minimal or no effort.

The issue of evidence is indeed problematic. Many researchers have advocated that the nurse keeps a record of all significant events which constitute the problem, from verbal/physical contacts, phone messages, emails – indeed all contacts.[7,31,32] This diary of trouble can go a long way in eliciting the problem. Often in such situations, healthcare workers have failed to compile such a dossier, either from a belief that it will be of little use or that such incidents will seem trivial, but this likewise puts them at a disadvantage in presenting their case.

The overall perception then from bullied nurses and healthcare workers is that management as a whole handles bullying situations very poorly. Not only do their immediate line managers in many instances fail to act, or act inappropriately, but general management in trusts and human resources departments come in for continued criticism. There is again both a general lack of understanding, and a reluctance to act at all managerial levels. Frequently victims in healthcare complain about:

- frustration and delay in dealing with bullying complaints
- issues being sidelined or ignored
- avoidance of dealing with bullying or not seeing it as that
- problems with lack of evidence (e.g. lack of record, or physical evidence)
- paying lip service to established policy.

Towards resolution: bullying in the light of organisational negotiation

Often when bullying investigations and formal hearings take place, conflicts manifest. In many instances, victims are left at a distinct disadvantage in their attempt at obtaining satisfactory redress. This can be particularly destructive where situations of unequal power predominate and powerful, often managerial groups begin to impose their definition of events. A classic example of this is Munday's study of manipulation of bullying events by deliberate abuse of policy within the educational sector (K Munday, personal communication, 2004). Munday examines how this was accomplished by liberal 'interpretation' of established disciplinary procedure. Negotiation is skewed predominantly in favour of the bully and, in Munday's own words, 'thereby ensuring the likelihood of justice is significantly diminished'. Such strategies involve organised groups, be it clique groups, nurse managers, general management or unions, etc., all of which may have vested interests and varied agendas.

The victim may feel very isolated from such group cohesiveness, even when they have had the confidence to take action. Those who are involved in negotiations and have the power to negotiate organisational goals may well cloak their own interests in terms of wider collective organisational goals to influence negotiations. Indeed, we see this by the rule bending and lack of decision in the dubious handling of many bullying hearings. Rule bending and manipulation can take many forms, from the hiding of patients' notes and subsequent altering of them (as in one case by a midwifery manager to set a victim up to fail) or, as in Mary's case, faking a letter of complaint about her.

We can now raise a number of points in relation to bullying negotiations in healthcare, all of which require consideration when dealing with bullying events.

- Victims are frequently at a disadvantage when formal negotiations take place.
- Manipulation of the negotiative context by the manager or others with vested interests is always a possibility – either to maintain the status quo or to forward their own agendas.
- Such interests may be cloaked in organisational legitimacy.
- We should be aware of the power differentials in such situations.

In many ways, and not unlike many large-scale UK organisations, the end result of bullying investigations within the NHS is frequently unsatisfactory to all concerned, but with the most trauma affecting the victim. These effects can be devastating. Quite apart from the overall negative health effect of bullying while the event is in progress, the implementation of the process of investigation takes its own toll. What is more worrying is that the effects of both prolonged bullying and investigation remain particularly traumatic.

An initial breakthrough regarding the length of these effects was noted by Leymann and Gustafsson in Sweden, where it was found that 95% of victims were suffering from post-traumatic stress disorder.[29] Importantly though, these victims did not suffer from the normal acute reactions of this disorder, but the situation was being constantly renewed *after* the bullying had ceased. Victims have a pervasive fear of being victims again, but also suffer from severe 'rights violations' that continue to affect their self-esteem and psychological and physical health long after the actual events. They may well manifest evidence of post-traumatic embitterment syndrome due to perceived massive injustice, and thus prove particularly difficult to help. Such violations are seen in, and compounded by, the inadequacies of the NHS in its approach and conduct towards bullying.

The net result is often a problematic outcome to interaction. In part such is the complexity of the situation that not all contingencies can be taken into account or established rules applied, and it is further compounded in bullying investigations by problems of continuity of investigation and momentum. It has been a continual theme throughout my research that it is the bully's manipulative actions that remain central to such issues. Once this is realised, then the bullying event can be tackled. The bully in particular is likely to use resources that remain most effective to their aims. If these involve secrecy, persuasion, manipulation and confusion, all creating conflict and disarray, then so be it. Such manipulation will be found throughout the bullying event.

References

1   Lewis M. *The social organisation of bullying in nursing: the accounts of clinical nurses and nurse managers.* PhD thesis. Manchester: Manchester Metropolitan University; 2003.
2   Randall P. *Adult Bullying: perpetrators and victims.* London: Routledge; 1997.
3   Sheehan M. Workplace bullying: responding with some emotional intelligence. *International Journal of Manpower.* 1999;20:56–69.
4   Liefhooge APD and Olafsson R. Scientists and amateurs: mapping the bullying domain. *International Journal of Manpower.* 1999;20:39–49.
5   Raynor C and Hoel H. A summary review of literature relating to workplace bullying. *Journal of Community and Applied Social Psychology.* 1997;7:181–91.
6   Einarsen S. Harassment and bullying at work: the review of the Scandinavian approach. *Aggression and Behaviour.* 2000;4:379–401.
7   Field T. *Bully in Sight.* London: Success Unlimited; 1996.
8   Raynor C. Theoretical approaches to the study of bullying at work. *International Journal of Manpower.* 1999;20:11–15.
9   Einarsen S, Raknes BI and Matthieson SB. Bullying and harassment at work and their relationships to work environment quality: an exploratory study. *European Work and Organisational Psychologist.* 1994;4:381–401.
10 Brim OG. Personality development as role learning. In: Iscoe I and Stevenson HW (eds) *Personality Development in Children.* Austin: University of Texas; 1960: pp. 127–59.
11 Leymann H. Mobbing and psychological terror at workplaces. *Violence and Victims.* 1990;5: 119–26.
12 Waller W. *The Sociology of Teaching.* New York: Wiley and Sons; 1961.

13 Burke K. *The Rhetoric of Motives*. New York: Prentice Hall.

14 Raynor S. *Bullying and Harassment at Work: summary of findings*. Stoke-on-Trent: Staffordshire University Business School; 2000.

15 Hinton D. The burgher and the villein: rethinking the problem of bullying. *New Era in Education*. 2002;83:51–62.

16 Petri H. Courting injustice: legal and moral issues surrounding workplace bullying. *New Era in Education*. 2002;83:57–62.

17 Sutton J, Smith PK and Swettenham J. Bullying and 'theory of mind': a critique of the 'social skills deficit' view of anti-social behaviour. *Social Development*. 1999;8:1.

18 Glaser B and Strauss AL. *Awareness of Dying*. New York: Aldine Publishing Company, Hawthorne; 1965.

19 Emmerson RM and Messinger SL. The micro-politics of trouble. In: Plumer K (ed.). *Symbolic Interactionism*, Vol 2. Aldershot: Edward Elgar Publishing; 1991.

20 O'Connell P, Pepler D and Craig W. Peer involvement in bullying: insights and challenges for intervention. *Journal of Adolescence*. 1999;22:437–52.

21 Hennesey D and Spurgeon P (eds). *Health Policy and Nursing. Influence, development and impact*. Basingstoke: Macmillan; 2000.

22 Handy CB. *Inside Organisations*. London: BBC Books; 1990.

23 Witz A. *Professions and Patriarchy*. London: Routledge; 1952.

24 Moloney MM. *Professionalism in Nursing: current issues and trends*. Philadelphia: JB Lippincott Co; 1986.

25 Davies C. *Gender and the Professional Predicament in Nursing*. Buckingham: Open University Press; 1995.

26 Benson KJ. Organisations: a dialectical view. *Administrative Science Quarterly*. 1977;18:13–16.

27 Pollitt C. *Managerialism and Public Services*. Oxford: Blackwell; 1993.

28 Traynor M. *Managerialism and Nursing: beyond oppression and profession*. London: Routledge; 1999.

29 Leymann H and Gustafsson A. Mobbing at work and the development of post traumatic stress disorders. *European Journal of Work and Organisational Psychology*. 1996;5:251–75.

30 Department of Health. *Zero Tolerance Initiative Campaign to Stop Violence against National Health Service Staff*. London: Department of Health; 1999.

Chapter 4

A case study approach

David Bullivent and Terry West

Introduction

In this chapter the objectives are to:

- briefly overview the national NHS perspective
- consider how this perspective filters down through organisations and to individuals
- examine different levels of experience in the workplace
- reflect on actions taken at organisational and individual level
- reflect on actions that could/should have been taken at organisational and individual level.

As we have seen in previous chapters, bullying is a complex and detailed process, and this process in the NHS appears to be similar to other situations in many large-scale organisations.

This chapter is purposively focused on real-life scenarios that originated from a national survey looking at workplace relationships. By the use of case studies based on real reported situations, we will provide a framework from which you can develop your own practice. Each scenario is different, and the intention is to broaden your knowledge so you more clearly recognise and understand the complex problems related to workplace bullying. Suggested strategies for action are provided, in order to encourage a way of thinking about situations. These, along with guidance offered in other chapters, should provide you with a comprehensive approach to workplace bullying.

View from the top

The Healthcare Commission NHS National Staff Survey for England tested staff opinion in the NHS over a variety of areas, reporting initially early in 2004 and for a second time early in 2005. Every NHS trust (acute, primary care, ambulance and mental health) took part in the surveys. All staff working in organisations with fewer than 750 employees were sent a questionnaire (a census approach), but in organisations employing more than 750 staff a random sample completed questionnaires.

In the survey, staff were asked if they had experienced physical violence, harassment, bullying or abuse from patients, clients, relatives, managers/supervisors or colleagues in the last 12 months. Results from the two surveys are broadly similar. In the report, 16% of staff said they had experienced physical violence, harassment, bullying or abuse from other staff and 27% from patients or their relatives. Further questioning revealed that staff who said they had experienced harassment, bullying or abuse reported it on 52% of occasions. When staff were asked if they felt their employers took effective action against such incidents, about half thought they did, with the rest saying they did not know how their employer would react. A number (12%) thought their employer would not take effective action if staff were bullied, harassed or abused.

The following draws on some of those scenarios from those who reported workplace bullying in the survey.

Case study 1: whole-organisation experience

> This is a large primary community trust (PCT) in the south of England, employing 800 staff on a number of different sites.

A large PCT received the results of the 2004 NHS national staff survey early in 2005 and was disturbed to find that 16% of their responding staff had said they had experienced harassment, bullying or abuse from staff in the previous 12 months. The report also highlighted the fact that the organisation was in the worst 20% of PCTs nationally for harassment, bullying and abuse. There had been a history of bullying in one department in the organisation, but management felt that this had been dealt with some years ago and the situation should have improved.

Options and action

Those working in the trust at senior management level quickly recognised that there was not a 'do nothing' option, not only because there was a moral commitment to improve the situation but also because there was the reality of the need to improve the position before it was remeasured in the next survey.

Short-term actions were proposed for the initial thrust and included:

- staff being encouraged to report all incidents
- staff being made aware of zero tolerance approach
- reported incidents to be reviewed by the most senior management team
- an investigation of trends
- provision of better support to staff and effective debriefing.

The trust recognised that much of the action relied on communication from staff, in particular a higher level of reporting of incidents, so action could follow. Good communication with staff was therefore crucial to change previous poor practice; initially this was in the form of open access focus groups, newsletters and notices.

The trust adopted a zero tolerance approach to bullying, which resulted in many staff thinking that bullying would be completely eradicated. In reality it has to be accepted that bullying will probably always be a feature of working life, but with a zero tolerance approach its nature and prevalence can shift.

What appeared to be emerging within this PCT was that:

- staff had concerns that they were prepared to voice in a *confidential* survey

- staff were not always prepared to report incidents when they happened
- staff were reluctant to become involved in a meaningful dialogue with managers or others in the organisation about how to improve the situation.

There are many reasons why this may be the case, and some suggestions of what might lead to reduced confidence in management and unwillingness of staff to be involved in finding a way forward are included later in this section.

In such a scenario as the above, ways to effectively manage workplace relationships include:

- using external agencies to build confidence, provide expertise and avoid tunnel vision
- looking closely at internal responsibilities and relationships.

External agencies

An external agency such as the Andrea Adams Trust can provide invaluable support to NHS organisations in terms of both general advice and the provision of an employee assistance scheme. In this case an external agency has been approached to provide expertise direct to the trust including:

- harassment and bullying training
- a mediation service when required
- policy review and implementation guidance.

In addition a totally confidential telephone helpline can be offered, with counselling if required, at a level of guaranteed confidentiality that can never be matched by internal arrangements in an NHS trust.

Responsibilities

The trust also implemented a vision for good practice in responsible working with staff throughout the PCT. This covers areas including harassment and bullying, and personal staff responsibilities are made clear. These responsibilities are conditional on the trust being able to achieve certain objectives on behalf of the staff.

For example, the trust may state 'In creating a caring, healthy supportive working environment, the trust will ensure that all employees are not routinely intimidated, harassed or bullied within the working environment'. Staff for their part must agree that they have a responsibility 'not to intimidate, bully, harass or victimise others'.

This approach has already been adopted as good practice in several organisations. It is important to note that the message clearly conveyed to staff is that the trust can never achieve its objectives unless the staff themselves take some personal responsibility, which can become part of appraisal, recruitment, policy-making and operational procedures. Drawing these strands together may help to build a confident relationship between the organisation and its staff.

Case study 2: the junior manager's experience

Graham is a 35-year-old ex-army non-commissioned officer (NCO) who joined the NHS in the mid-1990s. He was appointed as a junior manager in a computer department in a large acute trust.

Name	Graham Green
Age	35 years
Type of organisation	Acute trust
Profession	General management
NHS service	2 years

When Graham was interviewed for his first junior management post he was enthusiastic about a new career within the NHS. When offered the job, it was made clear to Graham that he was second choice: the person who was initially offered the post declined it. When Graham took up post shortly after the interview other members of staff repeated this information to him, including those who were in junior positions.

Early into the job, Graham's line manager commented that they would have been better off employing someone with more experience. This comment was repeated by other members of staff, particularly when Graham sought any help, advice or support in relation to his many new duties. Slowly other members of staff who had initially been sociable, particularly in meal breaks, seemed to find other things to do which did not include Graham. At the same time there seemed to be an increase in informal and minor complaints about Graham's performance, and accusations of his poor interpersonal skills and relationships.

Following the departure of a junior colleague who was not replaced, Graham made an unsuccessful attempt to obtain support from the line manager. Graham also approached the occupational health and human resources (HR) departments for support, but this was not forthcoming. Graham's health deteriorated under these pressures and he suffered a short period of sickness. As the situation did not change, Graham decided to resign rather than return to the workplace.

The conflict that often arises in situations of bullying is determining whether workplace bullying has occurred. In this scenario, Graham certainly felt that he had been subject to bullying in the form of inappropriate and unacceptable behaviour. This included:

- staff being aware that Graham was second choice – this could be seen as a form of public humiliation especially when more junior members of staff were aware of this fact
- the gradual decline of sociability of work colleagues meant that Graham gradually became excluded, ignored and marginalised
- informal and minor complaints about Graham's performance
- the non-replacement of a junior colleague left Graham in a situation where additional and more menial tasks were imposed, making targets more difficult to achieve and leaving Graham being set up to fail.

The poor response received by Graham from the occupational health and HR departments exacerbated his situation, and in this case, as in many cases, Graham chose resignation as the best solution rather than challenging the perceived unacceptable behaviour. This is understandable, but in itself means that workplace behaviour will remain unchanged and the wider workplace remains oblivious to the difficulties and problems being faced by some members of staff.

What could/should Graham have done?

- Contacted a mentor who could provide guidance and support.
- Contacted a harassment and bullying advisor (if available) in the trust.
- Joined a trade union and asked them to intervene.
- Delegated menial tasks to someone more junior to him.
- Sent a formal letter to occupational health and HR detailing his concerns/issues.

What could/should other managers/colleagues have done?

- Supported Graham in his request for help from occupational health and human resources.
- Covertly/anonymously reported the bullying to a senior manager in another department.

What could/should the employer have done?

- Contacted Graham during his period of sickness to ascertain the reason for it (occupational health or HR).
- Arranged to conduct a return to work interview which might have reassured Graham that they were prepared to listen to his concerns and take action.
- Conducted an exit interview facilitated by a manager from another department.
- Reviewed the dynamics of the department and made adjustments to the team roles.

Case study 3: the community nurse manager

Tina is a community nurse who has made rapid progress through various management training programmes. She was appointed as a community nurse manager heading up a six-strong team.

Name	Tina Jones
Age	27 years
Type of organisation	PCT
Profession	Community nurse
NHS service	4 years

In a PCT a new young community nurse manager, Tina, was appointed, having been fast-tracked into management and having shown a high level of management competence through distinctions in a regional training programme. Colleagues were initially impressed by Tina because of her efficiency, but later became concerned with the changes she made to their ways of working.

These changes meant that staff were required to attend more and more meetings, team briefings and discussion groups which were promoted by Tina as 'involving' the team members. However, time spent at meetings seriously decreased the amount of time for direct patient care, but case loads were not reduced to take account of this. Although Tina constantly requested input from the team members, any ideas put forward were quickly and publicly discounted by her. Generally then, Tina's agenda would be taken forward unopposed.

The question in this case is whether Tina is simply being an over-zealous and efficient manager or is she bullying the members of the team she has been brought in to manage?

- The requirement for the whole team to attend additional meetings with no reduction in workload will lead to targets not being met and will impede work performance. In fact it may also be setting staff up to fail in their duties.
- Conduct at the meetings is of concern. At one level, discounting the ideas of staff demonstrates typical bullying behaviour of overruling, ignoring and excluding. The fact that this was done in a public setting would also lead to a level of public humiliation for those who presented their ideas.

Here again we only have a brief glimpse of a scenario caught probably at an early level of concern. It may be that Tina considered herself to be dynamic and wished to implement changes quickly. However, whatever her intention, her behaviour can be considered to be bullying and will very quickly have a physical and psychological impact on the individuals in the team. Unchecked, the situation for the team will deteriorate rapidly, and within the team certain individuals may be particularly vulnerable.

What could/should Tina have done?

- Been receptive and aware of how the team worked.
- Considered team dynamics and effective team working.

What could/should other managers/colleagues have done?

- Taken collective action in the meetings and supported appropriate suggestions put forward by individual team members.
- Formally advised Tina that attendance at too many meetings was detrimental to patient care.
- Collectively sent apologies and not turned up for some/most of the less relevant meetings.
- Taken their concerns to Tina, and if unsuccessful then to her line manager.

What could/should the employer have done?

- Arranged an away-day for the whole team so they could bond and learn to work together.
- Offered Tina relevant training courses on team dynamics and team working.
- Ensured that the problem was satisfactorily resolved – often in the NHS the problem is 'solved' by moving/promoting the person causing the problem to a post in another department.

Case study 4: contract cleaner

Jemima is a contract cleaner in a large acute hospital. She is from Eastern Europe and has a basic understanding of English and finds it difficult to express herself.

Name	Jemima Dimitrov
Age	32 years
Type of organisation	Acute
Profession	Cleaner
NHS service	12 months

Jemima was a hospital cleaner employed by a contractor who provided cleaning services to a large acute hospital. Jemima started cleaning because her English was poor as she had only recently arrived from an Eastern European conflict zone. Jemima had been in this job for about a year and enjoyed the independence of having a set routine to follow on a day-by-day basis and took great pride in the quality of her work. She was not well known to her colleagues, managers or those who benefited from her work, as she preferred to keep a low profile.

A new secretary was appointed to a consultant in the hospital and they shared a small office suite. The secretary would run her finger over high surfaces while Jemima was working and would sneer or 'tut' to herself. Jemima did not react in any way to this. On one occasion the secretary and the consultant (who had always previously kept himself to himself when Jemima was cleaning) were talking when Jemima entered the office. The secretary jumped up and flew towards Jemima waving her hands saying: 'You can't clean now, surely you can see we're doing important work that must not be disturbed'. Taken aback, Jemima left the cleaning on that day. This then became a regular pattern whenever the consultant or in fact anyone else was in the office with the secretary. Jemima never spoke to the secretary and would simply leave the area. On future visits, comments and gesticulations from the secretary became more intense and regular.

After some months of this treatment Jemima found it more and more difficult to go to work, culminating in her taking a week off for what the doctor described as depression. On returning to the hospital she was confronted by her manager who advised her that he had received complaints about her work, understood that she had not been carrying out all her duties regularly and cautioned Jemima. As Jemima could not express herself fluently in English, she could not adequately explain the situation with regard to her particular problems, and because she misunderstood the nature of the manager's caution, she assumed that she had been dismissed and left the premises.

In this scenario is the secretary being over-enthusiastic in her job and trying to create a good impression in front of peers and senior managers? Or could her action and attitude towards Jemima be perceived as intimidation and bullying? How much of the situation has been caused because the secretary and/or the employer do not respect diversity and recognise other people's needs?

- Certainly the behaviour towards Jemima is typical of bullying: by her actions (running her finger over surfaces looking for dust) the secretary is criticising Jemima's work non-verbally.
- The secretary is sabotaging/impeding Jemima's work performance by not allowing her access to the office during her routine so that the cleaning can be done. The secretary may be setting Jemima up to fail in her job.
- The physical action of waving hands, gesticulating and making sudden moves towards Jemima is felt to be intimidating and could also be perceived as threatening.

What could/should Jemima have done?

- Informed her line manager about her difficulty in accessing the area to be cleaned. If necessary, Jemima should have asked a colleague/friend/advocate with a better command of English to speak on her behalf.
- Asked her line manager to agree with the consultant and secretary set times for their office to be cleaned, regardless of whether or not they are holding a meeting.
- Requested that her manager agrees standards of work with her and makes it clear the channels to follow for expressing any dissatisfaction with her work.

What could/should the secretary have done?

- Recognised Jemima's language difficulties.
- Understood that Jemima was working to a schedule and been more tolerant in allowing access to the office.
- As common courtesy, she should have spoken discreetly to Jemima if there was good reason for her not to clean at that time.
- If there was regular difficulty in access/performance, the secretary should have discussed this with Jemima's supervisor.

What could/should the trust have done?

- Ensured there was a close supervisory relationship with cleaning team members.
- Provided an opportunity for individuals to express themselves in one-to-one meetings with line managers. This omission should have been picked up during the appraisal process.
- Use advocates/interpreters when necessary.
- Outlined staff rights and responsibilities at induction.

- Ensured an appropriate structure was in place with the contractors to make sure Jemima could perform her job satisfactorily. This may have identified that Jemima was clearly having problems in a particular area, and an investigation should have been triggered.
- Conducted an exit interview with an advocate/representative present which might have avoided Jemima leaving the organisation thinking she had been dismissed. The trust might have retained Jemima as an employee and saved the expense and effort of recruiting a replacement.

Case study 5: senior consultant

Gerald Edwards is a senior consultant in a large acute hospital. His patients are often 'outliers' which means they can often be on several wards spread throughout the hospital.

Name	Gerald Edwards
Age	54 years
Type of organisation	Acute
Profession	Consultant
NHS service	27 years

Gerald is a senior consultant in an acute hospital who has to regularly deal with his patients being 'outliers' in general wards throughout the hospital, and quite often on one particular ward. (An outlier is a patient who is temporarily located on a ward with patients from other specialties due to lack of space on a designated specialist ward.)

After completing ward rounds in his normal work area, Gerald has to cross the hospital and fit in his round of outliers prior to dealing with other commitments. Inevitably the difficult scheduling causes Gerald considerable frustration. The ward rounds are usually less than ideal, and frustrating for both the nursing staff and Gerald. After the rounds Gerald often speaks to the ward sister in her office and as the door is often ajar his loud criticism of nurses can be heard by many people. A typical comment could be: 'The nurses are **** and don't know what they're doing. If you don't sort them out, I'll make sure they're sorted out'. These regular unpleasant exchanges lead to the majority of the nursing staff 'disappearing' when Gerald comes on to the ward and a grapevine is set in motion of what Gerald has done or said on that particular visit. When this issue is raised by nursing staff in ward meetings the ward sister says: 'Oh that's just his way and the consultants are under so much pressure here'.

Gerald is clearly frustrated by his working pattern, resulting in him displaying typical bullying behaviour, whether it is intentional or not. Bullying behaviour is portrayed because Gerald is:

- verbally degrading staff in a public venue

- threatening to take action if they do not perform as he wants
- intimidating the ward sister by threatening to go above her to get her staff disciplined
- intimidating members of staff because they are afraid of what he might say or do.

Although being a victim of Gerald's behaviour, the ward sister is also complicit in the bullying as she is not confronting Gerald and taking action against him through appropriate channels. By saying 'That's Gerald's way', the ward sister can be viewed as condoning Gerald's behaviour, and in doing so she is not supporting her staff against it. It is likely that patient care is also detrimentally affected as nurses avoid contact with Gerald on his ward round.

What could/should Gerald do?

- Take action with senior management to reduce the amount of outliers he is responsible for and discuss the possibility of increasing the number of beds on his specialist wards.
- Discuss his general issues with the ward sister in a meeting chaired by a manager able to give impartial advice.
- Find ways to reduce his other commitments to reduce the level of pressure he is under.
- Recognise the impact he has on other staff.

What could/should the ward sister do?

- Discuss her issues with Gerald in a meeting chaired by a manager able to give impartial advice.
- Take a training course on assertiveness so she is able to deal with Gerald more confidently.
- When Gerald criticises nurses she should ask for specific examples and defend her nurses if the criticism is unwarranted. She should also take issue with her nurses if their action is unprofessional/unsatisfactory.
- Advise her line manager of the situation and/or seek advice from the human resources department or her line manager.

What could/should the trust do?

- Offer opportunities for staff to attend personal development courses.
- Provide training for staff who may have to work with conflict and tension in their everyday practice. This might include assertiveness training, dealing with difficult situations, and conflict resolution.
- Help Gerald to work more efficiently and effectively by reviewing the organisation of provision for his patients.
- Ensure that interprofession difficulties are explored as part of the appraisal process, and resolution of difficulties forms part of the objectives in job plans.

Case study 6: outpatient nurse

> Marion is an experienced ward nurse who has worked on internal rotation for many years, but due to a family commitment has changed jobs and is now based in a busy specialist outpatient department.
>
> | Name | Marion Burton |
> | --- | --- |
> | Age | 42 years |
> | Type of organisation | Acute |
> | Profession | Nurse |
> | NHS service | 20 years |

Marion is an experienced ward nurse who has recently obtained a nursing role in a busy specialty outpatient department. Due to the nature of the work in this particular outpatient department, the nursing staff have to obtain a considerable amount of information from the computer system prior to and during patients' attendance. The system is complex, and totally different from the system Marion previously used. All staff working in the outpatient department have had training on the computer system. However, because the department is busy and there is a relatively high level of sickness, Marion has been told that there is no training available in the short term, and so she will have to 'pick things up as best she can'.

In the first few days of the new job Marion found that she was unable to keep up with or obtain all the information required by the computer system to ensure the efficient running of the department. Marion had to regularly ask colleagues to help, but as they were already under pressure this resulted in them finding the information themselves by quickly clicking across the keyboard and through the various screens, but they did not spend any time showing Marion how to do it. Marion therefore became increasingly frustrated, as did her colleagues who felt that their own duties were interrupted. The senior nurse in the area, supported by other colleagues, started to allocate or direct Marion to duties that did not necessitate obtaining information from the computer system. These duties included getting staff refreshments, running errands and acting as a chaperone. This became increasingly frustrating for Marion, who was used to working as a core part of a professional team.

Although this scenario is the result of unfortunate circumstances, the lack of consideration by colleagues of Marion's situation could be construed as bullying:

- withholding work-related information, albeit unintentionally – Marion cannot get the information she needs to work effectively so it could be said that she is being set up to fail
- areas of responsibility are being removed and menial tasks imposed, which affects Marion's professional status and ability.

Processes should be in place that allow individuals to:

- talk to people about their concerns/problems
- make sure people understand what is going on and what is expected

- negotiate different arrangements and support when things are not progressing to plan
- train for changing and different roles as required for effective service provision.

What could/should Marion do?

- Discuss her problems with colleagues and talk about how they are affecting her.
- Offer to do the training in detail at a mutually agreed time.

What could/should the department do?

- Set up adequate training as part of the induction process for newcomers to the department.
- Offer to train Marion at a mutually agreed time.
- Allow Marion to 'shadow' a colleague until she is familiar with the system.
- Revisit Marion's experience and provide opportunities for her to perform duties that are appropriate to her experience and level of skill.

What could/should the trust do?

- Investigate why there is an elevated level of sickness in the department.
- Ensure that staff receive adequate induction and training before performing specific duties.
- Ensure all staff have an appraisal early in their new roles and an appropriate personal development plan in place.

Summary

Case studies in this chapter have shown some ways in which bullying behaviour is manifested in NHS organisations. Examination of these case studies allows us to consider bullying from a number of angles: how it may emerge in terms of behaviours, how individuals may become aware of it, and how it may be handled within the NHS. Where interventions and actions are suggested these are by no means comprehensive, but they do help reveal the complexities inherent in real-life situations.

The next section identifies basic requirements for all trusts. Core policies should be available in every NHS organisation, along with support from occupational health and human resources managers who are present in most NHS organisations.

As part of standard procedures NHS organisations should have the following in place.

Exit interviews

In areas with high staff turnover, exit interviews in particular can reveal useful information as long as the leaver can be assured that their openness will not affect their future career. To obtain the best results, consideration should be given to having an experienced practitioner, unconnected to the leaver's work team, conducting the exit interview. The organisation should have a mechanism to collate the results of exit interviews and to consider whether the organisation or individuals within it have contributed in an inappropriate way to the leaver's decision.

Back-to-work interviews

Normally back-to-work interviews are carried out by line managers following sickness or absence. If the absenteeism is not an isolated and short event, it may be prudent for this interview to be carried out by occupational health, HR or a manager from an unconnected part of the organisation. If bullying was a factor in the absence from work it may well be that the line manager is either the bully or complicit with the bully, and therefore the problem will continue unnoticed by the wider organisation and remain unresolved if there is no 'external' involvement.

Whistle-blowing policy

The purpose of a whistle-blowing policy is to encourage staff to raise a matter when it is a concern, rather than waiting to be able to prove it has become an issue. A trust whistle-blowing policy helps all members of staff raise their concerns about bullying at an early stage and in the right way. The policy should aim to support staff and reassure them that if they raise a concern they will not risk losing their job and they will not experience any form of retribution. In addition, if staff act in good faith it should not matter if they are mistaken. The policy must also guarantee to respect confidentiality if staff request this.

Absenteeism policy

Absenteeism should be continually reviewed so that hotspots can be identified. Although this information does tend to be collected, generally little is done with it because of competing priorities and lack of time. In smaller organisations where HR capacity is limited, the use of specialist HR tools can monitor patterns of absenteeism. Through a scoring mechanism it is possible to identify trends in individual behaviour which can then be followed up with closer scrutiny.

Recruitment and retention

Organisations tend to collect detailed information about recruitment and retention. High levels of recruitment to particular teams/positions and difficulties in retaining staff are not only costly for organisations but may well indicate an unhealthy culture in the workplace. The organisation should have expertise in the understanding and investigation of this information, and the capacity to effectively analyse and investigate likely causes/issues where there is a shift away from the organisation norm.

Mentors

A robust mentorship programme for most members of staff can be extremely beneficial. Mentors tend to be selected from further afield, are unlikely to be influenced by local management, and with the trust of the individual can often open new avenues of problem solving if difficulties exist or emerge. Good mentors are also more easily able to objectively review an individual's concerns and confirm or refute the interpretation of the situation that has been portrayed.

Harassment and bullying advisors/investigators

Drawn from the workforce and often trained by external consultants, the harassment and bullying advisors can be very useful, particularly if they are taken from a cross-section of staff. These advisors should:

- be available to any member of staff on demand
- be trained to listen to the complainant
- talk through the issues
- help the complainant decide what action to take
- NOT take any active role in challenging identified bullies.

Staff charter

Staff charters are a useful way to confirm not only the trust's stance, but also the employee's responsibilities. The following is a sample of how a typical agreement might read:

> In creating a caring, healthy supportive working environment, the trust will ensure that all employees are not routinely intimidated, harassed or bullied within the working environment.

This is demonstrated by:

- respectful behaviour and professional working practices
- protection against bullying, harassment, victimisation, violence or aggression
- action on all reported incidents of intimidation, bullying, harassment, victimisation, violence or aggression
- the development and implementation of appropriate policies and procedures
- positive action taken on outcomes of staff opinion surveys.

In respect of this responsibility, the trust's targets are to:

- continually challenge all forms of intimidation, bullying, harassment, victimisation, violence or aggression within the trust
- raise awareness of issues
- provide external confidential support and advice.

> In creating a caring, healthy supportive working environment, all employees have a responsibility to not intimidate, bully, harass or victimise others.

This is demonstrated by:

- not practising or condoning any form of intimidation, bullying, harassment, victimisation, violence or aggression
- reporting any concerns or incidents of unacceptable behaviour
- supporting colleagues who have encountered intimidation, harassment, bullying, victimisation or physical/non-physical assaults
- showing respect for the diversity and culture of other staff and service users.

Finally

Staff should be encouraged to ask themselves:

> 'is there anything that:
> - I do
> - someone else does
> - the organisation does
>
> that means someone could be subject to, or feel they are subject to bullying behaviour?'

The organisation can therefore use a variety of informal and formal procedures and processes to identify and understand areas for concern. On collecting and collating all this information a picture will very quickly emerge that will enable the organisation to target its resources more effectively in order to reduce the negative effects of workplace bullying.

Reference

1 NHS National Staff Survey. Healthcare Commission. Accessible on http://www.healthcare commission.org.uk/NationalFindings/Surveys/StaffSurveys/fs/en?CONTENT_ID=4014131 chk=r62T4B

Chapter 5

Student nurses' experience of workplace relationships

Cheryl Hume, Jacqueline Randle and Keith Stevenson

This chapter outlines the concern that exists about bullying of students while they are gaining experience in the NHS. By drawing on our research with nursing students, we identify common issues that healthcare students generally are likely to face while undertaking clinical placements. In doing so we hope that any healthcare student on placement will be able to recognise if they are being bullied, and will become more aware of the options open to them on how to deal with it. We also hope that employers, clinical colleagues and educators reading this chapter will be made more aware of the actions they can take to support students.

By the end of this chapter you should be able to:

- be aware of the vulnerable position students find themselves in, due to the hierarchical nature of healthcare
- recognise the options open to students, should they decide to take action against bullying.

Evidence described in earlier chapters of this book shows that a culture of bullying exists in the NHS. We assume that healthcare students in clinical placements will be affected by this. Indeed previous work has shown that students:

- are often ignored[1]
- are personally criticised[2]
- are abused[3]
- receive inappropriate feedback[4]
- experience a decrease in self-esteem that leaves them depressed, anxious and powerless[5,6]
- are less likely to provide good clinical care[7,8]
- are likely to leave their course.[9]

In previous chapters we have seen that the abuse of power is a key element of bullying. Often students find themselves on the receiving end of bullying tactics, simply because they are on the 'lower rungs of the ladder'. The misuse of power and the vulnerable position students find themselves in have been well documented.[10,11] This misuse of power may be subtle or extreme, as seen in Alavi and Cattoni's description of how nurses would send student nurses to carry out observations on patients who had recently died.[12] In another case, Daiski describes nurses using students as personal slaves, and uses the example of qualified staff sitting at the nurses' station while students struggle to carry out the work on the ward.[13]

A longitudinal study carried out by one of this chapter's authors has shown that over the three-year training period, nursing students experienced qualified nurses exercising power over them and bullying them, often with them being ridiculed or humiliated in front of others.[5,6] Sometimes it was more subtle in nature, but still caused students to feel powerless and their self-esteem to be diminished.

This extract shows the extent of the problem:

> I wouldn't do it over again, no, not this. If I knew what it was going to be, I don't know, but I definitely wouldn't do this again. I never thought nurses could be so bitchy. I'm a grown woman and they've made my life hell really. My daughter's at school and she's had less bullying than me. They're just bullies, to other nurses and to the patients as well. They ought to be sacked.

Another student exemplifies her experiences:

> You were a waste of time as far as the staff were concerned ... I didn't think they could all be that bad, but then I realised what they were like. That's what worries me about going up to X; it's the staff that have the problems, not the patients. I'm the kind of person who'd like to say something but I don't think you can. It depends what ward you're on. I don't get upset, I just get annoyed and I can't ignore it. I can't go to bed annoyed, 'cos I can't sleep and then I wake up even more annoyed. So I think I'd have to go and speak to someone, someone above them without sounding too much that I'm telling tales. There's something that has to be done to get it sorted out to see why they're being this way with me.

These extracts, along with others in this study, strengthen what earlier chapters have identified, in that victims often experience negative physical and psychological reactions to bullying. These include:

- sleeplessness
- anger
- anxiety
- worrying
- stress
- self-hatred
- powerlessness
- decrease in confidence
- increase in absence/sickness
- intention to leave the job/profession.

By the end of their three-year course, students often described how they exhibited symptoms of burnout, apathy, passive anger and using distancing approaches to patients and colleagues.[5,6]

Additionally, although they had initially been horrified at the bullying practices displayed by some staff at the start of their course, they had come to accept that this was normal:

> Oh, but you just have to fit in and get on with the work really. The patients don't mind, so long as they get treated, that's all they're bothered about. Honestly, everything's fine.

It was not only students that were on the receiving end of bullying. Some students had witnessed patients being bullied. In the following scenario a staff nurse had refused a learning disability patient her money, because she did not approve of what the client wanted to buy. The student who witnessed this explained how it made her feel:

> I felt that it was Heather's money and that she was a grown woman who came across as knowing what she wanted. I felt she was being treated like a child just because she had a learning disability. If the staff nurse had just given Heather the money she needed and not even asked what Heather intended to buy, this incident wouldn't have happened.

A more severe example of bullying can be seen in the following extract, where an elderly male patient accidentally spills his used urinal in his bed. The student had to clean the patient and change his bed:

> I thought he was absolutely disgusting. He was horrible. He shouldn't have done it, and I think he just did it to draw attention to himself. I've never seen a man naked other than my husband ... I just keep avoiding him now. I've asked if I can work with another team and I can't wait for him to be discharged. I spoke to my mentor about it because I don't know if I should be feeling like this, but she said he was disgusting as well. He's still trying to get my attention and keeps trying to say 'hello' but I just ignore him.

There may be many different explanations for the above scenario, but it is important to note that the patient received inadequate care, and was placed in a vulnerable and humiliating position. The staff nurse mentioned appeared to collude with the student by agreeing that the patient was indeed disgusting. This was not a 'one-off' situation, and students routinely described events where they had been encouraged to participate in inadequate care to the detriment of the patient.

We can see, then, that for healthcare students, bullying can be problematic and recent prevalence studies such as the ones carried out by UNISON and the Royal College of Nursing (RCN) have shown the extent to which there is a culture of bullying in the NHS.[14,15] This has detrimental affects on staff as well as patient care. The research we have cited points to a culture of bullying in healthcare organisations that can adversely affect students' self-esteem and consequently their ability to provide patient care.

Reflection
From the extracts drawn from interviews with two cohorts of nursing students we can see how students can often be placed in a precarious position, simply due to their student role. We see also how it can have detrimental effects, not only on the student but also on the patient. The above scenarios were gained from one-to-one interviews conducted with approximately 70 students during a three-year period 2000–2002. Were these findings typical and generalisable?

An opportunity to answer this question arose in 2004–2005 when we conducted a specially designed survey on work placement experiences of a sample of student nurses in another school of nursing in another part of the country. In this survey second- and third-year students from a large school of nursing at a UK university were asked to identify the frequency and particular types of bullying behaviour they had experienced in their last clinical placement.

The survey

The survey was based on the questionnaire tool developed by Professor Lynne Quine used in studies that had looked at the extent of bullying experienced by healthcare professionals.[16,17] Permission was granted to use Quine's 'workplace bullying' questionnaire and adapt the wording where appropriate to fit the experience of nursing students. For our study, it was felt that the questions needed to be balanced out to ensure that students could report positive as well as negative workplace experiences.

We decided to select out the questions that had relevance to clinical placements for nurses, and provide a question style that would allow respondents to answer in a form that indicated that the behaviour:

- never happened
- happened only occasionally
- happened frequently, or
- happened a lot.

This format gave students the opportunity to answer each question about bullying behaviour in terms of whether they did or did not experience it and to what degree.

It was also felt that students should be given the opportunity to describe and explain their answers and, therefore, questions exploring what the student nurses felt about the negative experiences and what they had done about reporting them were provided for this purpose. To establish if students in particular branches of training experienced more bullying than others, or whether age or previous experience influenced responses, information concerning these issues was asked for at the beginning of the questionnaire. The questionnaires were distributed to 400 second- and third-year nurses who agreed to take part in the survey.

Was the sample representative?

The sample of returned questionnaires (313) was 78.3% of the number issued. Demographic variables of the students who returned questionnaires were compared to national percentages to assess how representative the sample was of the national student nurse population (*see* Table 5.1).

The most recent national figures were taken from data supplied by the NMC,[18] dated March 2005. However, it should be noted that figures supplied by the NMC are for trained nurses, as student data are unavailable. The comparison shows that the sample was a reasonably accurate reflection of trained nurses with the exception of the study described here having fewer mental health students and more child branch students.

In the study reported here, diploma students made up 76.7% of the respondents, and 23.3% of students were studying on the degree programme. The exact breakdown of figures in the study appears in Table 5.2.

Table 5.1 Comparison of demographic information from student survey returns with national percentages[18]

Demographic variable	Student survey returns (%)	National figures (%)
Female	92	91
Male	8	9
Adult branch	77	72
Child branch	15	11
Mental health branch	6	14
Learning disability	2	3

Table 5.2 Demographic breakdown of survey respondents by sex, age, course, and branch of training

Variable	Percentage
Number of respondents – 313	78
Sex	
male	8
female	92
Age (years)	
17–24	62
25–34	22
35–44	12
45+	4
Type of course	
2nd year diploma	49
3rd year diploma	28
3rd year masters	11
4th year masters	12
Branch	
adult	77
mental health	6
child	16
learning disabilities	2

What were the results?

Fifty-three percent (53%) of student nurses had experienced one or more negative interactions during the course of their placement. This figure can be compared with existing research on bullying in the qualified nursing profession. Quine, using the Workplace Bullying Survey, found that 38% of staff in a community health trust had experienced one or more bullying behaviours in the last month.[19] In a later study she also found that 44% of qualified nurses had experienced at least one or more of the bullying behaviours.[16]

In our study there were a significant number of bullying behaviours reported, and the type of bullying varied in frequency. The most frequent form of bullying was the feeling of being 'frozen out' of the nursing team. The least frequent was the threat of actual physical violence. The overall average of reported experiences of bullying was 16%, and that includes a high of 34% who reported experiencing the feeling of being intentionally excluded, down to 2.5% who reported experiencing threats of physical violence. The six most commonly reported negative interactions experienced by this sample of students are listed in Box 5.1.

Box 5.1 The six most commonly reported negative interactions experienced by students

---

- Being frozen out
- Destructive innuendo
- Resentment
- Humiliation in front of other staff
- Efforts being undervalued
- Unwelcome teasing

One in four respondents identified six common negative interactions that they had experienced. The highest incidence was that of being frozen out and ignored, then destructive innuendo and criticism, resentment, humiliation, efforts being undervalued, and teasing. Four of these came under the category of threats to personal standing regarded as bullying behaviour from Rayner and Hoel's definition.[20] Studies on qualified staff show that they are more likely to experience destabilising behaviours such as shifting of goalposts and undervaluing of efforts.[16] However, nurses experiencing behaviours of unjustified criticism and humiliation, and being frozen out or ignored is commonly reported.[16,21,22]

The percentage of students that had experienced each negative interaction was calculated, and a line of comparison has been inserted at 16.6% (1 in 6 people) to show how the results compare to the frequency of bullying found in the RCN Working Well Survey carried out in 2002.[15] The results show that more than one in six students experienced 12 of the negative interactions, and six of the interactions were experienced by at least one in four of the respondents.

Other significant results

A summary table of significant results is presented in Table 5.3 and each finding from the table is now discussed.

The perpetrators of bullying were often doctors or healthcare assistants (HCAs)

Doctors have long been a dominant group in healthcare, and studies have previously reported how they often use their power negatively against young newly qualified nurses.[13] Interactions with doctors have been shown to cause newly qualified nurses to feel intimidated.[23] It is not surprising that students also identified similar encounters with doctors. However, studies have also shown that students also experience negative attitudes from experienced qualified nurses and also healthcare assistants.[24,25] These staff use a more passive approach to destabilising students' confidence by ignoring students, not allowing them opportunities to learn, and generally excluding them from the team. In the survey it was exactly this

Table 5.3 Summary table of questionnaire responses

Type of difference	Finding
Most cited perpetrators of bullying	Doctors, healthcare assistants
Type of qualification and number of incidents	Diploma students reported significantly more experiences
Type of branch training and number of incidents	Adult branch reported significantly more incidents than child branch
Age and number of incidents	Older students aged 35+ years felt more undervalued than those in a younger age group
Sex and number and type of incidents	Male student nurses felt more sexually harassed and suffered more inappropriate comments and jokes than female students
Number of incidents reported versus number of students taking action	53% reported experiencing bullying behaviour, but only 29% took action about it
Type of action taken	Most talked to their mentor or course tutor
Most frequently cited reasons for not taking action	• Not serious enough to make a fuss • Staff perhaps just having a bad day • It's part of the student experience • Placement short enough to put up with it • Don't want to jeopardise my evaluation from mentor

type of passive behaviour from HCAs that nursing students reported. These behaviours included lack of appreciation, lack of communication and not being given opportunities to learn.

Diploma students reported experiencing more discrimination on the grounds of race, sex and disability than the degree students

As the diploma course had a much larger intake it is probable that there were a larger number of students from different ethnic backgrounds and with disabilities in the diploma sample. Research has shown that there is still considerable discrimination within NHS nursing toward people from ethnic minorities and those with disabilities. The RCN Working Well Survey found that people from ethnic minorities and those with disability were more likely than others to experience bullying and harassment.[15] More than half of those from ethnic minorities in this study felt that the bullying was linked to their skin colour.

Diploma students experienced significantly more hostility than degree nurses

This finding contradicts research that suggests degree nurses will be viewed more negatively by nursing staff.[26] Some studies suggest that degree students will feel more confident and assertive compared to students on a diploma course.[27] Confidence and assertiveness can make a person less vulnerable to bullying, and it may be that this is why the degree student nurses in this study experienced significantly less hostility.

Students studying adult nursing experienced more negative interactions than those in child nurse training

In particular, behaviours that lead to destabilisation were more commonly reported by adult branch students. It is possible that differences in the structure of children's nursing in clinical areas provide a more supportive environment for staff and students, and this may account for fewer negative interactions. In paediatric areas there are traditionally better staffing levels, staff have more power, and there is better team working. These would all be instrumental in providing a less oppressive environment and hopefully less bullying. However, there is only anecdotal evidence to support these claims. Research into differences in ward culture and their effect on bullying would need to be carried out to explore this further.

Students over 35 years old experienced negative interactions significantly more than those under 35 years

The older students (35 years plus) experienced discrimination, hostility and teasing more than their younger colleagues. Studies have shown that older students often feel that trained staff treat mature students as if they were just out of school, and fail to acknowledge the value of the older student's past experience.[28,29]

Male student nurses indicated experiencing significantly more sexual harassment than their female colleagues

Although the number of male students in the sample was small, they experienced significantly more inappropriate jokes being made about them. Research suggests that though male nurses often experience advantages being a minority, they have struggled to cope with being accepted in a female-dominated profession.[30,31] Patients are often less accepting of male nurses and, combined with negative experiences with clinical staff, these are probably contributing factors in the general attrition of male student nurses.[31]

Fifty-three percent of the study sample indicated that they had experienced negative interactions; only 29% of the students took some form of action

This means that 24% of students in the survey (over 75 students) experienced bullying but took no action. These figures can be compared to those in studies on qualified nurses. Quine, reporting a study published in 2001, found that 69% of qualified nurses experiencing bullying had taken some form of action;[16] the RCN report in 2002 found that 77% of qualified nurses experiencing bullying had taken action.[15] Students taking action against bullying, therefore, accounted for a significantly smaller percentage compared to qualified staff. Reasons for this could lie in the transient nature of the student's time on placement, with no more than 10 weeks on most placements. This might mean that students may be unaware of which staff members to approach with problems, particularly if their mentor is the cause of the problem.[32] Students are also a group with very little power, so are less likely to challenge negative behaviour.[33]

Students indicated that talking to someone about the event was the easiest form of action to try and resolve their situation

In both Quine's survey of nurse experiences of bullying in 2001 and the RCN survey in 2002, the majority of qualified nurses experiencing bullying talked to colleagues or reported it to senior staff.[1,16] Students in our survey reported talking to members from both the educational and clinical arena; personal tutors and mentors were used most frequently. Students commented that they were not always happy with the result of the action taken. Those that had brought the bullying to the attention of their mentor were more likely to achieve some resolution.

Mentors were considered an important source of support for students in clinical placement

According to studies looking at the value of mentors, when students experience good supervision and mentorship they settle into the clinical environment and team more quickly.[32,34] Good supervision enables students to develop confidence, increase their knowledge and move towards their potential.[35,36] Good supervision is also vital in situations where conflict needs to be resolved.[24] For some, but not all of the students in our survey, mentors were providing them with the support and help they needed, especially when they experienced bullying. This suggests that the creation of a good mentor–student relationship is a key component in supporting students who experience bullying.

Reasons for not taking action

Students were asked to explain why they had not taken action over the incidents of bullying they had experienced. Reasons for not taking action varied, but included:

- their experiences were not significant enough to complain about
- it was felt that staff were 'just having a bad day'
- it was part of the normal student experience
- as the placement was short they could cope with behaviours within that limited time
- mentors would have to complete an assessment and therefore they did not wish to jeopardise their chances of success.

Reflection
Bullying is still part of healthcare culture, and frequently part of the student experience. As students are a relatively powerless group it is not surprising that so many experience bullying behaviours. The existence of a hierarchy in nursing has been shown to perpetuate bullying, and students are seen as being the bottom rung of this hierarchy.[1,37] This means that they are more than likely to experience bullying behaviours from senior members of staff. It is also suggested that in many areas of training there is a generational culture of nurse-to-nurse abuse, with older members of staff perceiving that junior members should be treated as badly as they were during training.[3] It appears that this socialisation into a culture of abuse begins in training, with students

nearing the end of their training already using bullying tactics against junior colleagues.[5,8]

Student nurses, like other healthcare students, use a number of strategies to smooth the process of professional socialisation and an important one is that of 'playing the game' and 'fitting in'.[38] In the 'fitting in' period, students will put up with things and try to make sure they don't 'rock the boat'.[38] Also the fear of 'more hassle' or bad evaluation stops them taking action, and it has previously been suggested that fear of retaliation is a significant factor in under-reporting of negative experiences.[39]

Solutions to negative clinical experiences

Students who had witnessed good nursing care were able to offer their own solutions to bullying in healthcare. Most of these solutions suggested have already been identified in the literature and are listed in Box 5.2.

Box 5.2 Experiences thought to be helpful to combat the effect of work placement bullying

---

- Working with friendly, helpful and supportive staff
- Good mentorship
- Being aware of what form bullying can take
- Being aware of strategies to combat the effect of bullying

These issues are now discussed.

Working alongside friendly, helpful and supportive staff is important to students and has a positive effect on their clinical learning and confidence[32]

When students feel cared for and supported, they feel they are able to provide better patient care.[40] It also enhances self-esteem, increases motivation to learn and affirms students in their choice of nursing as a career.[41] Being included in the team gives students the opportunity to learn and practise nursing skills within the safety of the team.[42]

Good mentorship

Students who had experienced positive placements often commented on the presence of a supportive and enthusiastic mentor. Effective support has been shown to increase students' ability to fit into clinical settings and to make the most of the learning experience.[34,41] Sharing knowledge and involving the student in decision making were important, allowing students to deliver care in partnership with their mentor.[1,35] Good supervision from a mentor ensures that students learn care delivery and how to relate to patients in a safe environment and with support.[34]

Students need to be aware that bullying exists and how to identify if they are being bullied; they should be encouraged to report any bullying experienced or observed

One method that has been suggested to increase students' ability to cope with bullying is assertiveness training. It is suggested that assertiveness can enable students to counteract bullying and have more power to effect change.[33] From this it would seem that assertiveness training should be included as part of the nursing curriculum.

Using existing strategies to tackle workplace bullying

The RCN has produced a document specifically for nursing students who feel they have experienced bullying and harassment.[15] It provides students with information on various options for action against the bullying.

If a student decides to take action it is helpful to them if they start by taking informal action:

- talk to people – friends, mentors, personal tutors, etc.
- talk to the bully and request that they stop
- keep a record of incidents and interactions with the bully.

When an informal approach has not been effective, the student may choose to take formal action in line with the trust's harassment and bullying policy. It is likely this will include the following points:

- you will need written evidence of the date and time of incidents, location, nature of evidence, your response and feelings, whether you took action and what this action was, the names and status of any witnesses
- you should have written evidence of previous attempts to informally resolve the situation
- you should take a representative with you to any meetings
- you should be prepared to provide a written complaint that should be registered formally with the organisation's representative – if you are studying at a university this may be the course director, head of school or human resources administrator
- you will need to be prepared to wait while the investigation proceeds.

Conclusion

We hope this chapter has raised the profile of the concern that exists about bullying of students while they are gaining experience in NHS workplace situations. By drawing on our research with nursing students, we have identified common issues that potential future healthcare students face while undertaking clinical placements. In doing so we hope that students will be able to recognise if they are being bullied and, if they want to take action, will be more confident in taking some of the options open to them described here. We hope also that employers, clinical colleagues and educators who read this chapter, along with the next chapter on the trainer's perspective on workplace bullying, will feel that they can support much better those students who need their help.

References

1 Cahill HA. A qualitative analysis of student nurses' experiences of mentorship. *Journal of Advanced Nursing*. 1996:24:791–9.

2 Randle J. The effect of a 3-year pre-registration training course on students' self-esteem. *Journal of Clinical Nursing*. 2001;10:293–300.

3 Farrell GA. From tall poppies to squashed weeds: why don't nurses pull together more? *Journal of Advanced Nursing*. 2001;35:26–33.

4 Begley CM and White P. Irish nursing students' changing self-esteem and fear of negative evaluation during their pre-registration programme. *Journal of Advanced Nursing*. 2003;42: 390–401.

5 Reeve J. *Past caring? A longitudinal study of the modes of change in the professional and global self-concepts of students undertaking a three year diploma in nursing course*. PhD Thesis. Nottingham: University of Nottingham; 2000.

6 Randle J. Changes in self-esteem during a 3-year pre-registration Diploma in Higher Education (Nursing) Programme. *Journal of Clinical Nursing*. 2003;12:142–3.

7 Andersson EP. The perspective of student nurses and their perceptions of professional nursing during the nurse training programme. *Journal of Advanced Nursing*. 1993;18:808–15.

8 Randle J. Bullying in the nursing profession. *Journal of Advanced Nursing*. 2003;43:395–401.

9 Royal College of Nursing. *Bullying and Harassment at Work. A good practice guide for RCN negotiators and healthcare managers*. London: Royal College of Nursing; 2005.

10 Garland A. Beware of the bully. *Nursing Standard*. 1999;13:65–7.

11 Duffin C. Anti-bullying toolkit helps staff to analyse behaviour. *Nursing Standard*. 2005;19:4.

12 Alavi C and Cattoni J. Good nurse, bad nurse ... *Journal of Advanced Nursing*. 1995;21;44–9.

13 Daiski I. Changing nurses' dis-empowering relationship patterns. *Journal of Advanced Nursing*. 2004;48:43–50.

14 UNISON. *Bullying at Work*. www.unison.org.uk/acrobat/13375.pdf

15 Royal College of Nursing (2002) *Working Well*. www.rcn.org.uk/news/pdfs/1778-Working Well.pdf (accessed 3 December 2005).

16 Quine L. Workplace bullying in nurses. *Journal of Health Psychology*. 2001;6:73–84.

17 Quine L. *Grampian University Hospitals Workplace Bullying Survey*. Canterbury: Centre for Research in Health Behaviour, University of Kent at Canterbury; 2000.

18 NMC. *Statistical Analysis of the Register: 1st April 2004 to 31 March 2005*. London: NMC.

19 Quine L. Workplace bullying in NHS community trust: staff questionnaire survey. *British Medical Journal*. 1999;318:228–32.

20 Rayner C and Hoel H. A summary review of literature relating to workplace bullying. *Journal of Community and Applied Social Psychology*. 1997;7:181–91.

21 Brennan W. I'm talking to you! *Emergency Nurse*. 1999;7:16.

22 McMillan I. Losing control. *Nursing Times*. 1995;91:40–3.

23 Jackson D, Clare J and Mannix J. Who would want to be a nurse? Violence in the workplace – a factor in recruitment and retention. *Journal of Nursing Management*. 2002;10:13–20.

24 Hart G and Rotem A. The best and worst: students' experience of clinical education. *Australian Journal of Advanced Nursing*. 1994;11:26–33.

25 Jackson D and Mannix J. Clinical nurses as teachers: insights from students of nursing in their first semester of study. *Journal of Clinical Nursing*. 2001;10:270–7.

26 Eaton N, Williams R and Green B. Degree and diploma satisfaction levels. *Nursing Standard*. 2000;14:34–9.

27 Harrison S. Degree vs diploma. *Nursing Standard*. 2004;18:12–13.

28 Glackin M and Glacken M. Investigation into experiences of older students undertaking a pre-registration diploma in nursing. *Nurse Education Today*. 1998;18:576–82.

29 Kevern J and Webb C. Mature women's experience of pre-registration nurse education. *Journal of Advanced Nursing*. 2004;45:297–306.

30 Cunningham A. Nursing stereotypes. *Nursing Standard*. 1999;13:46–7.

31 Stott A. Issues in the socialisation process of the male student nurse: implications for retention. *Nurse Education Today*. 2004;24:91–7.

32 Nolan L. Learning on clinical placement: the experience of six Australian student nurses. *Nurse Education Today*. 1998;18:622–9.

33 Begley CM and Glacken M. Irish nursing students' changing levels of assertiveness during their pre-registration programme. *Nurse Education Today*. 2004;24:501–10.

34 Spouse J. *Professional Learning in Nursing*. Oxford: Blackwell Science; 2003.

35 Griffith JW and Bakanuaskas AJ. Student–instructor relationships in nursing education. *Journal of Nursing Education*. 1983;22:104–7.

36 Hanson LE and Smith MJ. Nursing students' perspectives: experiences of caring and not-so-caring interactions with faculty. *Journal of Nursing Education*. 1996;35:105–12.

37 Begley CM. 'Great fleas have little fleas': Irish student midwives' views of the hierarchy in midwifery. *Journal of Advanced Nursing*. 2002;38:310–17.

38 Gray M and Smith L. The qualities on an effective mentor from the student nurse's perspective: findings of longitudinal qualitative study. *Journal of Advanced Nursing*. 2000;32:1542–9.

39 McKenna BG, Smith NA, Poole SJ and Coverdale JH. Horizontal violence: experiences of registered nurses in their first year of practice. *Journal of Advanced Nursing*. 2003;42:90–6.

40 Dillon RS and Stines PW. A phenomenological study of faculty–student caring interactions. *Journal of Nursing Education*. 1996;35:113–18.

41 Gillespie M. Student–teacher connection in clinical nursing education. *Journal of Advanced Nursing*. 2002;36:566–76.

42 Wilson-Barnett J, Butterworth T, White E *et al*. Clinical support and the Project 2000 nursing student: factors influencing this process. *Journal of Advanced Nursing*. 1995;21:1152–8.

Chapter 6

A trainer's perspective

Ian Grayling and Keith Stevenson

Introduction

From a training perspective, bullying is an inappropriate, unproductive and wholly unacceptable set of behaviours that are rooted in the bully's own insecurity and relative lack of ethical and social skills. Therefore the most effective training intervention would be to work directly with the bully themselves. Unfortunately, where the bullying behaviour has not been officially recognised – and relevant discipline procedures invoked – any intervention directed at the 'alleged' bully would be unwise for a host of legal and semi-legal reasons. There are perhaps two exceptions to this situation, namely:

- where the bully recognises a personal need for training – maybe on a broader 'personal development' front (e.g. communication and interpersonal skills) – allowing the trainer/mentor/coach to facilitate a change in behaviour
- where it is possible and appropriate to look at group/team behaviour, in a depersonalised way, challenging inappropriate behaviours, reinforcing ground rules that empower team members (potential victims), and developing alternative and more ethical ways of working collaboratively.

A far more likely scenario in 'bullying situations' is for the trainer to support the victim of bullying. This can be effective not only in enabling the victim to establish better coping strategies and countermeasures but also – because of the interactive nature of interpersonal behaviour – in modifying the behaviours of the bully.

This chapter will therefore explore a range of training interventions: principally those aimed at supporting the victim, but also those that may be directed at the bully or the work group in which bullying is, or may be, taking place. The information presented here is intended to be:

- a useful starting point for individuals seeking a better idea of how they can become more resilient and empowered in dealing with bullying behaviour
- a guide for trainers, mentors and coaches looking for ideas on how to develop effective anti-bullying training interventions.

As a final note in this introduction and in keeping with the points raised above, we have organised the interventions discussed in this chapter around three main headings, namely:

- working with the 'victim'
- working with the 'bully'
- working with teams and organisations.

> **Box 6.1** Terminology: bullies and victims
>
> The use of terms such as 'bully' and 'victim' is convenient shorthand, only. From a 'personal development' point of view, we avoid labelling people in this way, thereby inferring personal character or 'nature'. Rather, 'bullying' and 'victimisation' are seen as behaviours or processes which, although maladaptive on both sides, can nevertheless be changed.

Working with the victim

Learning styles

For some victims of bullying behaviour, gaining a better understanding of the causes and dynamics of bullying may represent the first stage of their re-empowerment, and create a more solid basis on which to build practical and personal anti-bullying strategies. Others may feel the need for some essential 'survival' tips and skills at the earliest possible point in order to re-establish a degree of confidence to cope more effectively with the situation.

The difference between these two groups may be a reflection of 'personal learning style' which, in broad terms, distinguishes those who need to learn about something first before trying it out, on the one hand, and those who learn better through early experimentation and reflection, on the other. Learning styles are well known to teachers and trainers, but often neglected in practice. They should nevertheless be uppermost in the minds of trainers and coaches whenever they start to engage with learners for the first time (*see* Figure 6.1). Learning styles came to prominence through the work of David Kolb[1] and laid the foundation of our current understanding of the processes of 'experiential learning'. Readers will be able to find a wealth of information about this topic using most internet search engines.

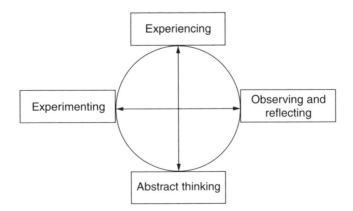

Figure 6.1 Kolb's learning styles.[1]

The essential point here is for the trainer to be aware when their chosen training method is not working for the particular individual concerned. For example, the trainer may want the person to practise assertive responses to verbal aggression. This will work well for someone whose preferred learning style is to try something out and to experience the result. Others may first need to see the technique demonstrated and then to reflect on it, and are therefore likely to resist immediate skills practice or fail to benefit from it. An awareness of different learning styles can help sensitise the trainer to the learner's needs and help them to adapt their coaching style accordingly.

The emotional impact of bullying

The experience of being bullied is upsetting, stressful and likely to impact negatively on the person's self-image and level of self-esteem. Repeated exposure to bullying may lead to feelings of helplessness and disempowerment, which in turn is likely to cause depression which can, as we know from the media, be life-threatening. The anxiety and distress caused by such experiences, coupled with the inevitable damage to self-confidence, can make it difficult for the person to take the initial steps towards a more constructive response to the situation. For this reason, it may be effective for the victim to access counselling prior to training.

Further information

Try an internet search on 'Learned helplessness' and 'Martin Seligman'.[2]

Counselling support

Counselling can be particularly effective in enabling the recipient of bullying to:

- express, and thereby mitigate, disabling emotions (anxiety, anger, frustration, etc.)
- obtain a more objective view of themselves, the aggressor/s and the circumstances surrounding the bullying incidents
- explore the possibility of personal change and re-empowerment through the development of new skills and ways of construing events.

Further information

Anyone wishing to acquire counselling skills that are particularly relevant to short-term, workplace interventions should read Egan (2002) *The Skilled Helper*.[3,4]

Counselling represents a fundamental tool for the trainer/coach and is firmly grounded on the underpinning skills of 'active listening' and empathy which are both discussed in more detail below, in the context of communication and interpersonal strategies for responding to hostility and bullying.

Other appropriate psychological support strategies might Include those designed to combat stress and anxiety.

Stress management

Techniques for managing stress are not easily described in a book of this nature and readers should consult the worldwide web or written sources for a comprehensive description or coaching manual. A quick search of the 'self-help' bookshelves or the internet will reveal a variety of techniques and approaches to combat stress, and many of these will be familiar to health professionals. When considering the available approaches, it is a good idea to match the technique, as far as is possible, to the personality of the person requiring the help. For example, it is unlikely that a highly extraverted individual will respond well to introspective visualisation techniques. Likewise, an introverted or shy member of staff may not favour aerobic exercise as a means of stress reduction. A further consideration in choosing an approach is to consider whether it is intended as an emergency – 'at the time' – technique, or one designed to reduce stress levels overall or minimise anxiety in future situations (*see* Figure 6.2).

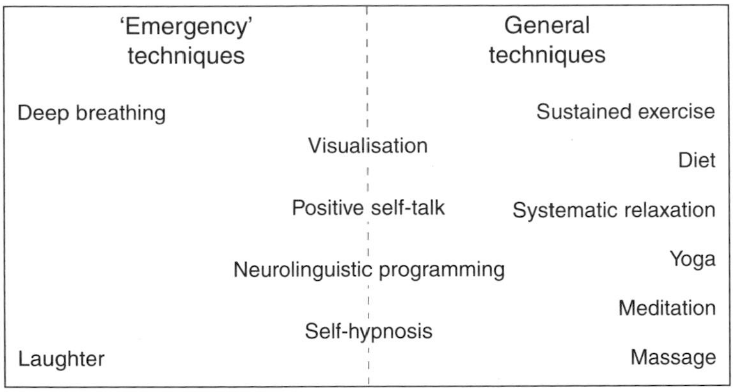

'Emergency' techniques		General techniques
Deep breathing		Sustained exercise
	Visualisation	Diet
	Positive self-talk	Systematic relaxation
	Neurolinguistic programming	Yoga
		Meditation
	Self-hypnosis	
Laughter		Massage

Figure 6.2 Stress management techniques.

Neurolinguistic programming (NLP) is currently a very popular approach to self-empowerment and life management. The empirical basis of NLP is, in part, questionable, yet practitioners and recipients of the techniques are, on the whole, complimentary about its beneficial and sometimes dramatic effect. NLP offers a range of techniques for stress and anxiety management as well as ones designed to boost confidence, self-esteem and interpersonal relating.

> **Further information**
> Check out books by Richard Bandler and John Grinder,[5,6] or carry out a web search on 'NLP'.[7]

For those victims of bullying whose learning style leads them towards a need to understand better and reflect on the circumstances in which they find themselves, an exploration of some of the psychosocial and organisational dynamics that can give rise to bullying may be helpful. Such a perspective is also most helpful in working with managers or teams to develop strategies that will help to prevent the abuse of employees in the workplace.

Understanding management and power

It is an accepted cliché, not without a degree of empirical support, that 'power corrupts'. Management, as it is traditionally understood, is a position of power and we must therefore be vigilant with regard to its potential abuse. While this is not, however, inevitable, certain conditions are likely to foster managerial abuse of power and its likely manifestation as bullying. Some of these conditions are:

- lack of, or inadequate, management training
- the absence of a strongly stated 'value base' promoting dignity and mutual respect at work
- inadequate procedures for dealing with abuses
- a culture of blame, distrust and insecurity
- a manager's lack of effective interpersonal and/or organisational skills
- poor communication, leading to a sense of isolation and distrust
- underperformance caused by lack of resources, clarity of purpose and poor co-operation
- stress.

Management style

In the late 1950s, Douglas McGregor surveyed the attitudes and beliefs that managers held towards their staff.[8] His research uncovered a range of beliefs on a continuum between two poles that he called 'Theory X' and 'Theory Y' (*see* Table 6.1). It is easy to see how managers holding beliefs that tend towards McGregor's Theory X may be inclined to a more controlling and potentially aggressive style of management.

Table 6.1 McGregor's theories X and Y

Theory X people	*Theory Y people*
• Are inherently lazy • Are self-centred • Are only prepared to work when this is unavoidable • Do not want or accept responsibility • Are resistant to change	• Are naturally inclined to work and enjoy it • Are self-controlled and internally motivated to work • Seek rewards in terms of self-esteem and sense of achievement and purpose • Are willing and able to direct personal effort towards a wider good

At much the same time as McGregor's publication of his Theories X and Y, two other researchers, French and Raven, proposed five different forms or sources of power commonly found in social groups and work organisations.[9] These are described below and are useful in understanding a possible link between management style and potential bullying behaviour.

> **Further information**
> See McGregor (1960) *The Human Side of the Enterprise.*[8]

- *Coercive power*: is the power to make others do something against their will, sometimes using physical as well as verbal and psychological threats. It is the form of power used by dictators and bullies and aims to ensure the compliance of others. In work situations, coercive power may take the form of withholding rewards, support, expertise or social inclusion.
- *Reward power*: is power based on the ability to issue or withhold rewards in return for compliance. This source of power can be ethical but also may be used in a coercive way.
- *Legitimate power*: this is power derived from 'role' or position within the group. French and Raven argued that monarchs, police officers and managers are all able to wield legitimate power. They noted, however, that legitimate power may be the acceptable face of less ethical, more coercive forms of power. An inherent danger with this form of power is that the person wielding it may forget that their power relates to their role and not to them personally.
- *Referent power*: this form of power comes from charisma and/or fame, and is the result of people wanting to be like, and to be liked by, you. People who are able to exploit referent power may find themselves using it for coercion.
- *Expert power*: is based on knowledge and skill that others require. It is a very common form of power, particularly in complex organisations built on clearly demarcated roles and multiprofessional working (i.e. the health service).

> **Further information**
> See French and Raven (1960) 'The bases of social power'.[9]

It is easy to see in French and Raven's analysis how power may be corrupt or become corrupting, creating the conditions in which bullying can take root and begin to thrive.[9] More recently, however, others have suggested the addition of a sixth source of power that arguably does not run the risk of corruption in the same way.

- *Enabling power*: is the power achieved – often unintentionally – through providing support and expertise to others in a way that enables them to achieve their goals more effectively and efficiently. This is a less obvious form of power (almost power by giving it away) that is achieved over a longer period of time, nurturing trust and leading to a sustainable, effective and ethical style of leadership.

Anti-bullying at work campaigner Tim Field has attempted to distinguish effective and ethical management behaviour from that which constitutes bullying.[10] He argues that 'bullying' is not the same as 'tough management' or 'assertive management'. The following excerpts are used with permission and aim to expose these two fallacies.

What some people call 'bullying' is really tough dynamic management
The purpose of bullying is to hide inadequacy. Good managers manage, bad managers bully. Bullies bully to hide their weakness and inadequacy, and to divert attention away from their incompetence. Many employers don't want to calculate the cost of low morale, poor productivity, poor customer service, high sickness absence, high staff turnover and·frequent grievance and legal action that are a consequence of 'tough dynamic management'.

Bullies don't bully, they're just being assertive
People who bully are unable to distinguish between *assertiveness* and *aggression*, and when challenged will speciously claim to be 'assertive'. Assertiveness, which is backed by integrity, recognises and respects people's boundaries and values, any request is polite and unconditional and there are no negative consequences if the person being asked says no. Bullies, who have no integrity, are aggressive, demanding, and regularly violate others' boundaries; aggression does not respect people's rights, and requests come with a negative consequence if the course of action demanded by the bully is declined.

(Tim Field[10])

Further information
The Field Foundation, PO Box 67, Didcot, Oxfordshire OX11 9YS, UK. www.bullyonline.org/workbully/manage.htm[10]

Management, leadership and command

The term 'management' appears to be gradually losing prominence in favour of 'leadership'. This reflects a gradual transition from a hierarchically organised and demarcated workforce, typical of the Industrial Age, towards flatter organisational structures with (largely self-managed) multiprofessional teams of the Information Age.

Management means, in its original sense, hands-on adjustment and control of a machine. During the Industrial Age, people were the 'means of production' requiring the co-ordinating control of managers. In the Information Age, workers are multiskilled, flexible problem solvers, with almost endless access to information and knowledge. The 'knowledge workers' of the 21st century need less management and more leadership to align and empower them in a common purpose set within a clear value base and agreed operational guidelines. From another perspective, this is a move from McGregor's Theory X to Theory Y.[8]

Set within this perspective, it is even more apparent that there is no place whatsoever for aggressive and authoritarian styles of management within the modern health service. Healthcare, of course, often includes 'emergency care', and for this reason there are times when leadership, in the modern sense, is not appropriate, and unambiguous, assertive command is what is required. But this is not 'bullying' even when crisis gives rise to frayed tempers and abrupt communications, possibly littered with colourful language.

Most writers on leadership, today, recognise that most people working in a management role need at various times to enact leadership, management and command roles. The trick, of course, is to know when each one is relevant. It is important to recognise that aggressive or bullying forms of coercion do not, and should not, feature in any one of these roles.

The UK health service, however, and particularly the secondary acute sector, retains a very traditionally managed and divisionalised type of organisation. Traditional, militaristic command and control management styles coupled with inter-professional barriers present a problem in a service that is expected, under current political thinking, to adapt itself to multiprofessional and cross-boundary working in support of a seamless flow of patient care. All of this is a potential source of stressful change and role ambiguity which needs to be carefully negotiated to avoid an otherwise likely 'human toll'.

Procedural strategies for victims

There are a number of practical countermeasures that victims of bullying can take to either minimise the incidence and impact of bullying or to support processes and procedures designed to deal with it. The trainer/coach can help the victim by suggesting these strategies and facilitating their development.

Antecedent causes and triggers

Victims need to consider carefully the circumstances in which bullying behaviour is being manifested. In what locations, times and situations is it most frequently occurring? Is it generally when alone with the aggressor or in certain company? Are there identifiable circumstances that tend to precede incidences? This type of analysis should help to:

- identify the antecedent causes or triggers to a bullying episode and then to consider how these can be avoided (if possible)
- predict occurrences and arrange for a witness to be present (or even to record the incident, in secret –with a dictaphone for example – for use in later procedures)
- plan and rehearse interventions at early stages of typical bullying episodes, in order to reduce the probability of escalation.

One way the trainer/coach can support the victim in this is to encourage them to maintain a reflective diary or log of events, which can then be discussed. A written record of this type is, of course, also invaluable in pursuing formal internal or external legal proceedings.

Assertive responses to bullying

A common strategy in combating bullying in schools is to teach 'at-risk' children a repertoire of assertiveness skills. Assertiveness skills are not, however, offered as an instant or total 'cure' for the problem – rather, they provide the child with an alternative strategy for responding to bullying behaviour in a way that maintains a degree of empowerment and avoids a negative loop of victim-like responses re-inforcing the victimising behaviour of the perpetrator. With adults, assertion skills have the potential to be wielded in a more sophisticated way and (hopefully) in a context in which the possibility of violence is less.

While bullying behaviour aims to weaken the recipient, assertive behaviour effectively undermines that purpose by substituting the expected compliance or effect with a controlled and empowering response. For someone who is already feeling disempowered as a result of bullying, having the belief and confidence to try out new behaviours will not, however, be easy. It is therefore important that the skills are developed at a comfortable pace and with frequent opportunities to practise in a safe environment before attempting them for real. For this reason, coaching and realistic role-play may be beneficial.

What follows is a basic introduction to some of the skills of assertion that can be usefully applied when working with the 'victim' of bullying. It is, nevertheless, only an introduction and readers should refer to the abundance of literature on the subject available through libraries and on the worldwide web.

Defining assertiveness

A quick internet search shows that it is easy to find descriptions of assertive behaviour. A typical example would describe assertive behaviour as involving:

- standing up for your own rights, while recognising the rights of others
- communicating accurately and honestly with others on an equal basis
- reaching our goals without preventing others reaching theirs
- giving ourselves and others credit for success
- allowing ourselves to make mistakes
- respecting our own needs enough to ask for what we want, and to say 'no' where appropriate
- dealing with issues while they are small
- respecting assertive behaviour in others.

Assertiveness *is not* aggressiveness or 'being bolshy' – neither does it relate mainly to women. Rather, assertiveness is 'grown-up' talking: it is how adults should relate to others (*see* Figure 6.3).

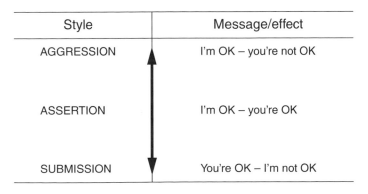

Style	Message/effect
AGGRESSION	I'm OK – you're not OK
ASSERTION	I'm OK – you're OK
SUBMISSION	You're OK – I'm not OK

Figure 6.3 The 'traditional shorthand' comparison of relationship styles.

The reality, however, is that communication between 'colleagues' is often dishonest for fear of the consequences of 'straight talking' or, at worst, through a misguided need to manipulate. Assertiveness is the sensible mid-ground between aggressiveness and submissiveness. It is not always helpful to use the term 'submissiveness' to describe the opposite of 'aggressiveness' because of the wider set of contexts in which the word is commonly used and, therefore, a broader set of connotations.

Current practice therefore favours the term 'non-assertive behaviour' to express the opposite pole. The original terminology is useful, however, in relating these two poles of behaviour to a well-known aspect of animal (humans included) behaviour: namely, the 'fight–flight' response. The fight–flight response refers to the behavioural response to threat and its physiological counterpart, adrenaline. In situations of stress or threat, animals may display either aggressiveness (fight) or submissiveness (flight), according to factors relating to the characteristics of the threat and the environment in which it is happening. The importance of this is that aggression (anger) and submission (fear) are products of the same phenomena – threat, stress, insecurity, etc. This is useful knowledge in understanding the nature of bullying and in dealing with it.

> 'All cruelty springs from weakness.' (Seneca, 4 BC–AD 65)

Assertive behaviour acknowledges the worth of the other person and, in so doing, has the additional benefit of helping the aggressor to deal more constructively with the insecurities that underlie their bullying behaviour. Effective assertion therefore incorporates a significant amount of 'empathy' ('I'm OK – you're OK'[11]) through a cyclical process of asserting and 'active listening' – previously called 'the broken record technique', although this metaphor is now somewhat outdated.

The assertion process

The process of asserting may start with the assertive message or it may start with empathy (*see* Figure 6.4). Why should we ever start with empathy? The answer to this is that sometimes we may be faced with overt aggression – possibly the threat of violence – in which case, the sensible option is to diffuse the tension in the situation through empathic listening, *before* telling the other person why they should not behave in that way: personal safety and security always come first.

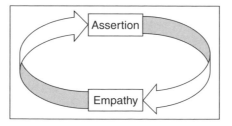

Figure 6.4 The process of asserting.

Delivering an assertive message almost always invites a defensive response from the recipient, and it is therefore extremely important that the trainer offers sufficient coaching to cover this eventuality. Defensive responses on the part of the person receiving the assertive message threaten to derail the whole process as our previous conditioning pulls us away from the assertive, adult-to-adult, style of communication and towards equally defensive or even aggressive responses on our part (*see* Table 6.2). This must be avoided if the assertion is to be effective.

Table 6.2 Examples of responses

Response	Analysis
A: 'When you call me stupid in front of patients, I feel angry because it makes me seem unprofessional and undermines the patient's confidence.'	Good assertive start
B: 'Well, I can't wait for you to get it right!'	Defensiveness
A: 'I'm still trying to learn and you're not helping.'	Assertion lost!

Defensive responses

The way to deal with a defensive response to an assertive message is to listen with empathy before restating the assertive message. It is important that the person who is asserting retains their poise by recognising and inhibiting their conditioned drive to argue. Instead they should substitute the alternative, and far more effective, interpersonal skill of 'active listening' (described in more detail, below). Defensiveness responses are likely to continue throughout the interaction, but continuing a cycle of listening and assertion will either gradually undermine the aggressor's non-assertive (yes, 'non-assertive') behaviour, bringing it to a manageable level, or will cause them to behave in an even more unreasonable fashion which they would find hard to justify to themselves or to others (*see* Table 6.3).

Table 6.3 Alternative responses with active listening

Response	Analysis
A: 'When you call me stupid in front of patients, I feel angry because it makes me seem unprofessional and undermines the patient's confidence.'	Good assertive start
B: 'Well, I can't wait for you to get it right!'	Defensiveness
A: 'So, my need to take time to get to grip with these new skills is creating difficulties for you?'	Active listening (empathy)
B: 'You might say!'	Still defensive
A: I would like us to talk more about that – however, when you call me stupid in front ... etc.'	Good assertive continuation

The assertive message

The example of assertion illustrated above utilises a principle or template for creating an effective assertive message known as 'The three-part assertion message' (*see* Box 6.2).

Box 6.2 The three-part assertion message

---

1 A specific and non-judgemental description of the behaviour to be changed: *'When you call me stupid in front of patients'*
2 An honest an accurate description of how you feel about it: *'I feel angry'*
3 An explanation of the tangible effect this has on you (or others): *'because it makes me seem unprofessional and undermines the patient's confidence'*

The words describing the three parts to this message are carefully chosen and should be studied carefully. The first part *must* be non-judgemental or it will run the risk of a valid criticism over the choice of words used. Consider for example, *'When you treat me like a xxxx'* in comparison with *'when you treat me without respect'*.

The second part emphasises the accuracy of the emotional impact. Compare, for example, *'I feel a little bit annoyed'* with *'I am incandescent'*. Delivering an honest and accurate statement of feelings requires what is now increasingly being called 'emotional literacy'. Although cultural variations occur, on the whole we are not taught or encouraged to articulate our emotions, with the result that our verbal repertoire is generally poor when it comes to describing emotional states. Improving emotional literacy is an important underpinning skill of assertion (and empathy) and involves collecting and rehearsing a wider vocabulary to express not only the different emotional states but also the relative strength of the experience (*see* Table 6.4).

Table 6.4 Emotional literacy (vocabulary)

Emotion	Weak	Mild	Strong
Anger	Bothered	Annoyed	Furious
Fear	Worried	Scared	Terrified
Stressed, etc.	Pressured	Wound up	Stressed out

These are examples only. A thesaurus is a good place to research an emotional vocabulary. It is important to develop a language of emotion that feels natural.

The final part of the assertiveness message is essential, and must not therefore be omitted. It makes clear to the recipient that there are unacceptable (by any code of conduct) consequences of their behaviour, giving them the opportunity to consider their behaviour in a more global and rational way. Failure to complete the statement with this explanation of consequence runs the risk that the message may be dismissed as a mere expression of feelings (or difference of opinion), rather than understood as a very real need to change.

Other aspects of assertive language

A relatively small adjustment to the choice of words used during an assertive exchange can have quite profound effects on both parties to the interaction. The following tips and examples should be practised in a range of situations so as to become part of the natural verbal repertoire when dealing with actual verbal aggression and manipulation.

- *Use 'I', not 'we', 'they' or 'everybody'*

A statement is more powerful (empowering) when it is made from the standpoint of 'I' rather than a hypothetical collective of others (we, they, everybody). Compare the following:

1   *'Everybody knows that this is not the right way to prevent infection.'*
2   *'I don't believe this is the right way to prevent infection.'*

Which of these two statements is more direct (honest) and empowering?

- *Change 'can't' to 'I don't want to'*

'Can't do' invites debate about capability whereas 'I don't want to' is – again – more direct, honest and therefore empowering. Expressing wishes in such an unambiguous manner will usually, however, require a follow-up statement to justify this stance.

- *Change 'should/ought' to 'could/might'*

Compare the following statements in response to a manipulative or unreasonable request:

1   *'Perhaps I ought to do this another way.'*
2   *'Perhaps I could/might do this another way (... if ...).'*

The first of these two statements imposes compulsion on the speaker, whereas the second maintains choice and the possibility of bargaining.

Changing the habitual use of language requires considerable practice. The trainer should therefore consider a variety of techniques to help reinforce the new patterns of verbal behaviour. These might include:

- direct coaching and role-play
- mental rehearsal
- maintaining a reflective log/diary of experience using the techniques.

The use of empathy in assertion

The relevance of using empathy in assertion was explained earlier. Empathy does not require us to feel sympathy for another person – which in the case of a bullying colleague or boss can be somewhat hard to achieve. Empathy is about trying to understand 'where the other person is coming from'. We can, and should, do this without having to feel either sorry for them or obligated as a result. It is counterintuitive, but nevertheless the case that empathy – whether we want it or not – tends to cause us to identify with the other person in ways, and at a level, that would be highly unlikely without it. If assertiveness is about us respecting ourselves as well as respecting others (I'm OK – you're OK), and if aggression is itself the manifestation of anxiety, stress and insecurity then a closer emotional affiliation with the aggressor may not be a bad thing.

Empathy is best described as a product of 'active listening' which is a process of actively trying to find the meaning in what another person is trying to express (often inadequately). It therefore extends far beyond the superficial 'hearing' of the other person speaking, typical of many everyday verbal exchanges.

Active listening involves several key techniques which, like the assertive statement, must be practised in order to develop the confidence and capability to use the skill in stressful situations. Typically, people find active listening very demanding when they initially attempt it, but then discover that it quickly becomes more natural and less tiring to maintain the level of concentration required for effective performance.

Paraphrasing

Paraphrasing involves reflecting back what someone has said to you but, as much as possible, in your own words. The purpose of this is to:

- help you ensure that you have interpreted the other's meaning correctly (and giving them a chance to correct any misunderstanding)
- show the other person respect (even if they are failing to show respect towards you)
- absorb and dissipate hostility.

A useful technique for paraphrasing is to preface the statement with an introductory clause such as '*So, what I think you are saying is ...*'. Good paraphrasing will have a significant impact on the interaction and, with consistent use, will cause the aggressor to moderate and even change their behaviour as they begin to realise that they are not achieving the expected response and, perhaps, the 'victim' is not the threat they thought they were. Further examples of paraphrasing are shown in Box 6.3.

Box 6.3 More examples of paraphrasing

- If I understand you correctly ...
- Can I just check that I've got what you are saying ...?
- I heard you say ... , did I understand you correctly?
- So, your view is ... , is that right?

Exploring with open questions

It may be necessary, and certainly useful, to explore the aggressor's position by probing it with open questions (*see* Box 6.4). The Greek philosopher Socrates invariably defeated his opponents in debate by the skilful use of questioning to expose the flaws in their arguments. This technique can be equally effective in challenging bullying and manipulative behaviour. It is at its most effective when coupled with paraphrasing to ensure that the meaning or intent underlying a statement is exposed and agreed. Consider, for example: '*You have said that you need to be hard on me because I'm new to the team – how is that helpful?*'.

Box 6.4 Open questions

Open questions start with:

- how ...
- what ...
- which ...
- when ...
- who ...
- why ...

Bullies do not like probing questions, particularly when questioned in a public arena. Questions such as the following can be rehearsed as a formulaic strategy:

- 'What is your evidence for what you are saying?'
- 'Who have you checked this out with?'
- 'What other solutions have you considered?'
- 'How do you know this is a problem?'

Empathic responses

Empathy is a powerful interpersonal skill because much of our behaviour is determined by underlying insecurities, aspirations and values. Bringing these undercurrents to the surface exposes hidden agendas, and enables a more constructive analysis of the real issues that lie at the root of difficult behaviours.

Empathic responses are a means of checking out the unexpressed emotional content behind the actual words spoken. The response must, however, be tentative – we can only ever guess what another person feels, and we may get that wrong. Empathic responses might therefore be considered as a speculative paraphrase focusing less on what was said and more on what was not said. For example:

> 'When you said that this is not how we do it in this practice, I got the impression that you felt anxious about me wanting to do things in the way that I was taught – is that correct?'

> 'Are you worried about that?'

While empathy exposes hidden agendas, it also shows concern, ensuring that the assertive interaction remains respectful and engenders a more constructive level of interaction.

Being prepared

It should be clear from the analysis of assertive techniques, so far, that effective assertion needs preparation and practice, although it is possible and desirable for the skills to become more spontaneous. There are two related strategies that are worth considering in the short term or until the skills are more embedded.

It may be necessary temporarily to withdraw – verbally or physically – from a bullying encounter, in order to spend time to calm down and prepare an assertive response or even arrange to have a witness to the planned interaction. Statements like those below can be useful in 'buying time':

> 'I am not prepared to talk to you about this right now. I want some time to think about this and then talk about it later.'
> 'I am feeling too angry to deal with this in a rational way right now, but I do want to deal with it later.'

Preparing to assert may involve time spent writing down and practising a three-part assertion message or a longer statement to preface an assertive interaction. An appropriate statement might start off along the lines of:

> 'I need to talk to you about the incident earlier and I would like you to hear me out before you comment. I will then try hard to understand your view with regard to the situation and will expect that we will be able to talk it over in a rational and respectful manner. I want to start by saying ... (insert three-part assertion message).'

Working with the bully

Establishing and directly addressing bullying behaviour by individuals or groups within organisations is never easy. If bullying has been unequivocally identified, it is essential that the health trust or its subsidiaries signals its disapproval, and discharges its legal responsibilities by formally addressing the situation through discipline procedures. However, discipline procedures are in themselves difficult to enact, requiring clear and valid procedures and staff who are confident and competent in carrying them out. Organisational procedures are frequently poorly enacted in such difficult circumstances, leading to the possibility of counteraction through the tribunal and wider legal systems. Effective training for all those involved is therefore essential.

It should be remembered that bullying behaviour may be rooted in insecurity and failure to develop more ethical and interpersonally effective behaviours, probably from an early age. From this perspective, 'bullies' may also be considered as 'victims' worthy of support and, if available and appropriate, counselling. *Supporting the 'bully' in this way does not imply or involve a 'soft approach'*. Outcomes of disciplinary proceedings are still upheld, and a commitment to support the individual concerned should in no way influence (i.e. reduce) the severity or stage of proceedings that has been reached as clearly defined by established procedure.

Where bullying is suspected but unproven, there are training interventions that can be invoked that do not explicitly label an individual and that offer them the kind of professional development opportunities that would be available in a more general context. These interventions may be effective in helping the 'erstwhile' or 'potential bully' to develop the new skills that will enable them to cope more effectively and to discover better ways of relating to and influencing others. Relevant training may include:

- assertion and active listening
- negotiation and ethical influencing
- building and managing high-performing teams
- leadership and management skills

- stress management
- time management
- change management
- anger management.

It should be noted, however, that attendance on training courses alone may do little to change behaviour. What is required is a more comprehensive and coherent solution whereby the intended outcomes of training are incorporated within internal performance management (appraisal) targets that are then properly evaluated through a range of potential measures that may include reflective practice, mentoring and/or 360° feedback. If readers are unfamiliar with any of these terms, they should consult a reputable and current text on human resource management or take advice from their HR department.

Working with teams and organisations

Conflict arises naturally in teams because it is rare for two or more people to share the same beliefs, interests, goals or preferred approaches to work. Conflict is therefore natural and inevitable and the purpose of conflict resolution is not to eliminate conflict – or to get rid of the people involved – but to handle it constructively even though it is, of its nature, uncomfortable and stressful.

According to Bruce Tuckman all groups or teams go through five typical stages of development, namely:[12]

- *forming*: team members attempt to establish roles, responsibilities and relation-ships
- *storming*: cliques and factions form, leading to conflicts
- *norming*: team becomes more cohesive and working relations become more established
- *perfoming*: the team functions well without the need for much leadership
- *mourning (or adjourning)*: Tuckman added this to the model at a later point – team members resist and react to the break-up of the group.

Further information
See Tuckman (1965) 'Developmental sequence in small groups'.[12]

There are two aspects of this model that may be relevant here. Firstly, Tuckman makes the case that conflict arises naturally as the team works through its differences and before it is able to function as a high-performing unit. We can assume that some of the behaviours exhibited in the team at this stage may be construed as bullying. The second aspect is less direct or obvious, in that once the team has developed a degree of coherence, new members may find it difficult to integrate into the group, being seen – at least in the short term – as outsiders.

Mobbing is a term used when bullying is by a group of people – effectively, ganging up – rather than by an individual. Typical behaviours include the group engaging in constant criticism towards the targeted person, gossiping about them, spreading rumours and false information or causing them to be isolated or ostracised from social contact.[12] Like other forms of bullying, mobbing may become more serious and frequent over time. Research by Jean Lennane identified 'whistle-blowing' as a major cause of mobbing in the health service and the *BMJ* continues to report periodically on similar cases of victimisation.[14]

Further information

See Leymann (1990) 'Mobbing and psychological terror at workplaces' and Lennane (1993) 'Whistleblowing: a health issue'.[13,14]

Another related dynamic is where the team composition is changing frequently, as for example in a teaching hospital. In such a situation it is easy to imagine the work group rarely progressing beyond the 'storming' stage. This sort of 'team' environment would undoubtedly be stressful due to a constant readjustment of relationships and responsibilities, and uncertainty with regard to the achievement of targets. In other words, there would be a fertile ground in which bullying and non-assertive behaviours can flourish.

Fortunately, there are measures that can be taken to combat the group-based dynamics that can drive aggressive behaviours. Implementing these measures requires a training intervention starting at the organisational level, involving senior and influential personnel within the service and filtering down to team leadership level. The aim of such an intervention must be to create a top-to-bottom culture that will not tolerate bullying and will deal with it wherever it occurs.

Creating an anti-bullying culture

A typical definition of organisational culture would be 'the pattern of shared beliefs, attitudes, assumptions and values in an organisation which shape the way people interact and influence strongly the way in which things get done'. Changing organisational culture is a tough proposition and there is not a great deal of consensus in the human resource literature on how this is most easily achieved. Cultures are created by people, nevertheless, and people are capable of change. From this perspective there are lessons from social psychology that can give some guidance as to how culture can be changed.

People generally prefer to behave in a way that is commensurate with their attitudes and beliefs. If you want a person to change their beliefs or attitudes towards something, one way is to make them behave differently. Anti-discriminatory laws and positive action have done much to change UK attitudes and beliefs with regard to diversity. For example, racist jokes, largely thought acceptable in the 1970s, are, on the whole, considered to be in very poor taste and wholly unacceptable nowadays. It is clear that forcing people to change their behaviour with regard to discrimination has gradually led to a cultural shift whereby values, beliefs and attitudes have moved in the same direction. From a psychological point of view, this can be explained by 'cognitive dissonance' which predicts that if an individual is forced to act in a way that is contrary to their self-belief or attitudes, they experience psychological discomfort which has to be resolved by changing their cognition or belief system.[15] Taking this as a basis, it can be argued that trying to change behaviour in an organisation by changing culture is likely to be less effective than trying to change culture by changing behaviours.

So how can we change behaviour in a way that creates an anti-bullying culture?

- An unequivocal mandate for change must be communicated from the very top to the very bottom of the trust. This message must be simple, clear and visibly championed by key figures within divisions, departments and/or professional lines of accountability.
- Behaviours that promote effective collaboration (*see* Box 6.5), high-performance team working and leadership need to be identified, monitored and evaluated.

Box 6.5 Collaborative behaviours at work

- Provided efficient and effective help (timely, appropriate, so the other person could succeed) to a colleague
- Exchanged needed information resources (no more, no less than required)
- Provided constructive feedback on a colleague's work (for the colleague's benefit)
- Challenged another's reasoning or conclusions (to solidify his/her point of view)
- Proposed mutually supportive action (to achieve tasks together)
- Influenced a colleague's efforts (to achieve an outcome that is better for both of you)
- Acted in a trusting way (with or toward another)
- Was motivated by, or motivated a colleague (to work together on a challenging assignment)
- Kept anxiety and stress in check (so that another could get on better unhindered by anger or fear)

Adapted from Johnson and Johnson (1989)[16]

In order to effectively monitor and evaluate collaborative behaviours, performance management (appraisal) systems need to work! This means real-time monitoring of meaningful – and fluid – targets, rather than infrequent and meaningless reviews of 'dead' targets. Performance management is not an occasional management function: *it is 'management'*.

Linked to the first point in Box 6.5, all teams and workgroups should be encouraged to commit to a fundamental set of ground rules that guide day-to-day collaborative working. These can be developed, and therefore 'owned', by team members themselves with some guidance. Any group of people will, if asked, come up with a set of conditions that they reasonably believe would maintain a (psychologically) 'safe' working environment capable of supporting collaboration and mutual support. Their list will probably be quite short, and will correlate most closely to the description of assertive behaviour listed earlier in this chapter. It is further likely that each of these ground rules will be underpinned by one recurring theme – namely, 'mutual respect'.

Other policies and (particularly) procedures need to be reviewed to ensure that they support a 'dignity at work' policy and dovetail neatly with it and each other.

Conclusion

It should be clear that a range of training interventions are available to combat bullying at the individual and organisational level. The extent to which these interventions can be deployed, however, will depend on the personal confidence and competence of the trainer/coach.

This chapter aims to provide an introduction to some of the concepts and practices that can add value in the fight against bullying and abusive behaviour at work. Trainers who wish to become more involved in this type of employee support should clearly strive for a degree of mastery in these areas beyond what is possible from reading this chapter alone. It is a fundamental principle that all teachers/trainers should be learners first. In this Information Age, the resources available for self-development are immense, and the trainer needs to exploit this.

The experience of many in-house trainers is limited to the delivery of formulaic programmes in the 'training room', and they may have neither the confidence nor the particular competencies to deal with individuals in a one-to-one coaching situation. In this particularly sensitive area of personal support, it is essential that the trainer also evaluates their own development needs against the nationally benchmarked *Standards for Learning and Development* which fully map the depth and breadth of understanding and skill necessary to facilitate individual, team and organisational learning.[17] (These standards are due to be superseded in 2007 by new teaching standards for the whole of the learning and skills sector.)

References

1   Kolb DA. *Experiential Learning*. Englewood Cliffs, NJ: Prentice Hall; 1984.
2   Seligman MEP. *Learned Optimism*. New York: AA Knopf; 1991.
3   Egan G. *The Skilled Helper*. Belmont, CA: ThomsonWadsworth; 2002.
4   www.gp-training.net/training/mentoring/egan.htm (accessed 5 December 2005).
5   Bandler R and Grinder J. *Time for a Change*. California: Meta Publications; 1993.
6   Grinder J and Bandler R. *Frogs into Princes – neuro linguistic programming*. Real People Press/UT; 1979.
7   www.richardbandler.com (accessed 5 December 2005).
8   MacGregor D. *The Human Side of Enterprise*. New York: McGraw Hill; 1960.
9   French JPR Jr and Raven B. The bases of social power. In: Cartwright D and Zander A (eds). *Group Dynamics*. New York: Harper and Row; 1960: pp. 607–23.
10 The Field Foundation, PO Box 67, Didcot, Oxfordshire OX11 9YS, UK. www.bullyonline.org/workbully/manage.htm (accessed 5 December 2005).
11 Harris T. *I'm OK – You're OK*. Tennessee: Avon Books; 1967.
12 Tuckman B. Developmental sequence in small groups. *Psychological Bulletin*. 1965;63:384–99.
13 Leymann H. Mobbing and psychological terror at workplaces. *Violence and Victims*. 1990;5:2.
14 Lennane K. Whistleblowing: a health issue. *British Medical Journal*. 1993;307:667–70.
15 Festinger L. *A Theory of Cognitive Dissonance*. Evanston, IL: Row and Peterson; 1957.
16 Johnson D and Johnson R. *Cooperation and Competition: theory and research*. Edina, MN: Interaction Book Company; 1989.
17 *Standards for Learning and Development*: see www.standards.dfes.gov.uk/learningmentors/nos (accessed 5 December 2005).

Chapter 7

Workplace bullying: reflections

Keith Stevenson

Why did I agree to help write part of this book? What did I hope it would achieve?

I agreed to help write part of the book because I felt that the book would be a valuable resource and tool for healthcare staff. For those who are either experiencing bullying or witnessing workplace bullying, I hope that they will benefit by having something they can consult which might help them understand what is happening to them or others. I hope the benefits will be that NHS staff reading this book will feel more able to combat workplace bullying.

Throughout the book, it is apparent that the term 'bullying' is a difficult term to define accurately. For the purposes of the book an operational definition of bullying is provided by Adams: 'the persistent demeaning and downgrading of people through vicious words and cruel acts'. Examples of what might be regarded as bullying behaviours are listed in early chapters. If, like me, you felt you thought you knew what bullying was I urge you to read through these chapters again and reflect on how persistent demeaning and downgrading phrases about you or your friends might begin to take effect. Until I helped to adapt questions for a survey on students' experiences of bullying in clinical areas, I did not appreciate the full breadth and depth of bullying behaviours that healthcare staff can experience.

The word bullying summoned up in me stereotypical images of physical intimidation linked to long-forgotten childhood schooldays. However, workplace bullying can be much more subtle than that, and its effects much more serious. One of the key points listed by Jacqueline Randle at the outset of this book is that bullying needs to be understood in context before it can be addressed. Just focusing on rooting out the bully through disciplinary procedures or just supporting the victim may not be sufficient. It's easy to build a mental picture of the typical tough bully and the typically weak and hesitant victim. As we are reminded in earlier chapters, the danger of these rigid stereotypes is that we begin to see the bully as nothing but a bully, and the victim as nothing but a victim. Examples of scenarios are given where it is apparent that the bully can also be a victim and vice versa.

The point that bullying does not occur in isolation but rather is linked to context and culture is developed by authors in later chapters. Keith Hickling's chapter (Chapter 2), for example, is useful in that it helps the reader shift their attention from just looking at the bully's behaviour to a broader perspective of how workplace environments can produce and sustain acts of bullying. He reminds us that the study of bullying in organisations has been fraught with difficulties and false trails that have concentrated on investigating attributes of the bully or attributes of the victim. If we wish to pursue an understanding of bullying, Hickling urges us to follow Scandinavian research that places the study of bullying within the organisational context. In this way, bullying is understood to be the outcome of at least four interrelated factors: namely, interpersonal, intrapersonal, organisational and social dimensions.

Hickling does not stop there either. He feels that correlational research suggests that bullying could also result from another interaction with a work context, producing stress stemming from role ambiguity and role conflict. While the evidence is correlational and not causal, the associations do seem to point towards such a relationship. Hickling completes his chapter with some useful advice on what to do if you experience bullying or are charged as a manager with preventing it happening or dealing with it effectively.

The view that bullying is a learned response mediated by the organisational structure of the NHS is developed by Malcolm Lewis (Chapter 3). Based on his interviews with managerial staff and staff who had experienced bullying, the picture of a 'situated serial bully' emerges. This approach attempts to help us see the bully not as a psychotic temper tantrum waiting to happen, but more as a calculating problem solver who uses bullying tactics to ensure activities occur in the way they want them to.

In Lewis's view, bullies can actually be seen as intentional actors manipulating their world to keep it they way they want it. This intentional manipulation may take time for recipients to recognise. The fact that bullying behaviour has been operational and 'normalised' for some time makes it quite difficult for the victim to suddenly challenge it and effect change, and this difficulty explains, in part, its insidious long-term effect.

Other factors contributing to bullying survival include failure to recognise the bully's activities as bullying, having a complaint redefined as a 'personality clash', and the blame for the problem then being rested on the complainer. Like Hickling before him, Lewis also points to the organisational structure in healthcare that supports managerial bullies. Power is exerted downwards in healthcare organisations. The culture of nursing is quoted as almost providing the perfect habitat for the manipulative bully. Lewis goes on to identify the powerlessness that infects the lower-status healthcare workers who are made to feel they have failed if they need to seek help in dealing with quite unrealistic managers' demands.

Lewis's chapter paints a depressing picture. Not only are healthcare workers bullied, they are bullied quite often by intention. The managerial healthcare culture openly admits to bullying as a viable technique for getting things done. To openly admit to using bullying techniques but to excuse them on the grounds that it is essential in getting staff to meet targets provides the opportunity for management to justify their actions. Provided the victim does not take action, the bullying can continue. Where victims finally take action, Lewis points to evasive strategies bullies then employ that deflect the charge, imply the victim is troublesome and more often than not leave the bully in the clear.

Is there any light at the end of this tunnel? Lewis is not overly optimistic. There is certainly a long way to go. The need for all levels of staff to feel that there is a clear communication route where what they say will be listened to, and that action will be taken quickly in response to a complaint are two key areas still seen by staff as stumbling blocks to the removal of management bullying behaviour in healthcare.

David Bullivent and Terry West, in Chapter 4, present a more optimistic view as they use the findings of a survey of bullying of qualified healthcare staff to provide the framework for a series of individual case studies. The case studies cover a wide range of contexts and styles of bullying behaviours. Each case is then discussed and actions that might be taken to break the cycle of persistent bullying are considered. This approach should be really useful to readers who recognise a particular situation's description as resembling their own. By reading the suggested courses of action that the authors provide, it is possible that a reader may take appropriate steps to bring the bullying they have been experiencing to an end.

Another optimistic message presented by Bullivent and West comes in the form of managerial structures and procedures that they feel will help identify persistent bullies within an organisation. They recommend exit interviews as well as interviews on returning to work after illness as a means of identifying the effect of individual managerial staff on employee sustainability. Encouraging whistle-blowing with safeguards built in, and keeping a close eye on absenteeism and the reasons for it are another two management processes that could help an organisation defend itself against the harbouring and concealment of bullies. An awareness of high staff turnover, and the reasons for it, may provide further clues to areas where staff prefer not to work. Specific assistance to bullied staff is also suggested with the role of trained mentors or trained harassment/bullying advisors who can support a victim and help them choose an appropriate course of action if it is thought to be necessary.

Finally, the idea of workplace bullying being addressed by organisations buying into and setting out a staff charter is refreshing. The charter is jointly produced by staff and management and sets out the principles of good non-bullying management. Importantly, it clearly states the willingness of management to support staff against any instances of bullying identified by staff, irrespective of their position in the organisation. A culture that supports victims would strip away the cover that those bullies need in order to operate. Creating a culture where management supports the workforce against bullying and is prepared to devise procedures that it is not frightened to implement suggests to me a definite way forward. I recommend this chapter to all managers who wish to remove bullying from their organisation.

I hope that readers will have found the final two chapters as interesting and informative as I did in researching and helping to write them. The first (Chapter 5) reports the findings of two surveys of students' experiences of bullying they experienced on work placement. Jacqueline Randle's work on the experiences of students as they progressed through a three-year training programme indicates that students' self-esteem decreases over time, even though their nursing skill levels are increasing. Her work also shows how a significant proportion of students felt angry at how their philosophy of care in nursing was not fulfilled in what they saw and experienced while on placement.

The chapter then goes on to show how the thoughts and feelings from student interviews carried out in 2000–2001 were also evident in the more recently completed large-scale survey of diploma- and degree-trained students in 2004–2005. The results of this survey identified the prevalence and nature of the most frequently reported bullying behaviours. Over half the students returning questionnaires (170) had experienced at least one negative behaviour, and almost one-third of the sample either experienced being frozen out or endured destructive innuendo or both. Students were reluctant to report bullying behaviours to their mentors, citing not wanting to 'rock the boat', or 'being prepared to sit it out' as the main reasons for not making formal complaints.

Students on placement are on the lowest rung of the organisational ladder and are therefore obvious targets for workplace bullying. The findings of this survey provide food for thought and suggest that students perhaps need to be better prepared for their placement experience, and given opportunities to practise the skills to help them benefit from, rather than just survive, placements.

The final chapter (Chapter 6) considers bullying from a trainer's perspective. It has the aims of helping individuals to become more resilient and empowered in dealing with bullying behaviour and to act as a guide for trainers, mentors and coaches looking for ideas on how to develop effective anti-bullying training interventions. The chapter draws on principles of human behaviour that have been established as 'tools to think with' over the last 30 years or so. In this respect the chapter suggests that trainers need to be aware of student learning styles and how they interact with adopting new ideas.

In a similar fashion, trainers need to be aware of the helplessness that bullied members of staff experience. Helping bullied staff explore their feelings of helplessness and begin to consider action requires a considerable number of counselling skills. Skills of empathic listening and non-judgemental support, for example, are crucial for trainers required to support staff who feel badly about themselves and their situation.

The trainer can support bullied staff and provide activities that mimic the difficult situations they currently experience or may experience in the future. Staff can be encouraged to act out possible solutions and these can be discussed and, if needs be, practised further. The skills of assertiveness may be helpful here and to that end there are some useful tips on expressing yourself assertively provided in this chapter.

The trainer, of course, may focus their attention on the bully and help them reflect on their interpersonal style and create a less manipulative operator. To this end, the trainer may be usefully employed in helping an organisation create an anti-bullying culture. Following on from previous chapters, the power of an organisation's culture is emphasised and the power for good that can be created when the organisation becomes focused on a non-bullying culture is reinforced.

The training chapter provides an introduction to some of the concepts and practices that can, if professionally delivered, help victims to begin to fight back against the bullies. The success of trainers in supporting individuals and helping them stand firm will depend on their skills and knowledge and commitment to the cause, and their confidence to work with individuals in this area.

I feel that this book provides food for thought and should stimulate reflection about bullying and its effect on workers in the NHS. I think anyone interested in finding out about bullying behaviour in the NHS and what they might do about it will be better informed after reading any or all of these chapters. If readers find the content helps them understand how bullying operates in the NHS it will have partly achieved its aims. If practitioners who have suffered bullying, or management who wish to dismantle a bullying culture, through whatever means described here, improve their lot and the lot of others then it will truly have achieved its aims.

Reference

1 Adams A. *Bullying at Work – how to confront and overcome it.* London: Virago Press; 1992.

Index

Employment Rights Act (1996) 23
encountering workplace bullying 20–1
exercises, workplace bullying 17–18
exit interviews, standard procedures 58–9
external agencies, case study 49

Field, Tim 9, 83

gender bias 41

HCAs *see* healthcare assistants
Health and Safety at Work Act (1974) 22–3
healthcare assistants (HCAs), student
    nurses 68–9

intent 9–10, 25–8, 98
inter-role conflict, role conflict 14
inter-sender conflict, role conflict 14
interactive approach 25–45
interviews, standard procedures 58–9
intra-sender conflict, role conflict 14
intraprofessional conflicts 41
investigators/advisors, standard procedures
    60
isolation 41–2, 43

junior manager's experience, case study
    50–1

key issues 2
Kolb's learning styles 78–9

leadership and command, management
    83–4
learning styles, trainer's perspective 78–9
legislation 22–3
Lennane, J 94
Leymann, H 94

management and power, trainer's
    perspective 81–4
management, leadership and command
    83–4
management styles 81–3
managerial control 37–40
managers, workplace bullying 19–21
manipulator 43–4
    bully as 29–30
measuring workplace bullying 15–17
mentors/mentoring
    standard procedures 59–60
    student nurses 72

Munday, K 38, 43
mutual pretence 36

Negative Acts Questionnaire (NAQ) 16–17
negative acts, workplace bullying 16–17
negotiation, organisational 43–4
negotiations 40–2
nurse manager, case study 51–3
nurse, outpatient, case study 57–8
nurses, student *see* student nurses

Offences Against the Person Act (1998) 22
open questions, assertiveness 90–1
options, case study 48–9, 51–61
organisational accounts, bullying 25–45
organisational adequacy, dealing with
    bullying 42–3
organisational bullying 41
organisational context, workplace bullying
    10–12
organisational issues 40–2
    policies and procedures 42–3
    power differentials 43–4
organisational negotiation 43–4
organisations/teams, working with
    93–6
outpatient nurse, case study 57–8

paraphrasing, assertiveness 90
PCTs *see* primary community trusts
personality, bullying and 26–8
person–role conflict, role conflict 14
policies and procedures, organisational
    issues 42–3
post-traumatic stress disorder 44
power and management, trainer's
    perspective 81–4
power differentials, organisational issues
    43–4
preparedness, assertiveness 91–2
pretence 31–2
    mutual 36
preventing workplace bullying 19–20
primary community trusts (PCTs), case
    studies 48–9, 51–3
procedural strategies, for victims 84–92
procedures and policies, organisational
    issues 42–3
Protection of Harassment Act (1997)
    22

questionnaire, NAQ 16–17